Activities Manual

for

Stress Management for Life
A Research-Based Experiential Approach

Michael Olpin
Weber State University

Margie Hesson
South Dakota State University

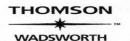

WADSWORTH

Australia • Brazil • Canada • Mexico • Singapore • Spain • United Kingdom • United States

Printer: Thomson/West

0-534-64478-3

Cover image credit: Getty Images/Martin Barraud

Thomson Higher Education
10 Davis Drive
Belmont, CA 94002-3098
USA

For more information about our products, contact us at:
Thomson Learning Academic Resource Center
1-800-423-0563

For permission to use material from this text or product, submit a request online at
http://www.thomsonrights.com.
Any additional questions about permissions can be submitted by email to **thomsonrights@thomson.com.**

Table of Contents

CHAPTER 1
STRESS IN TODAY'S WORLD

CHAPTER OUTLINE
Use this outline to take notes as you read the chapter in the text and/or as your instructor lectures in class.

I. **STRESS IN TODAY'S WORLD**
   A. Never before have college students been faced with such vast opportunities, such freedom of choice, and such an array of information.
   B. Yet these opportunities, these many choices, and this information overload can be the factors that leave you feeling overwhelmed and stressed.

II. **STRESS - WHAT IS IT?**
   A. Coming up with an accepted definition of stress is not easy.
      1. Stress, stressors, eustress, distress, good stress, and bad stress are all terms to describe the experience we know as stress.
      2. One common definition of **stress** is this: a demand made upon the adaptive capacities of the mind and body:
         a) Stress depends on your personal view of the stressor and can be both a positive and a negative factor in your life.
         b) It is your *reaction* to the events in life, rather than the actual events, that determines whether the outcome is positive or negative.
         c) Your capacities determine the results. Stress is a demand made upon the body's *capacities*. When your capacities for handling stress are strong and healthy, the outcome is positive. When you lack the ability to handle the demands, the outcome is negative.
   B. Stress can be stimulating and helpful.
      1. It can provide changes and challenges to push you along, to provide opportunities to learn and grow, and to provide the impetus for accomplishing your goals in life.
         a) We can relate managing stress to building muscle
            (1) The key is in finding the right balance. Too little weight will not produce the desired results; too much weight may result in fatigue and injury and will not produce the desired results.
            (2) You need to overload the muscle just enough so that it will become stronger.
         b) So it is with stress: too little stress leads to boredom and lethargy; too much stress leads to physical and emotional breakdown. The right balance leads to a productive, healthy life.

III. **YERKES-DODSON PRINCIPLE**
   A. Harvard physicians Robert Yerkes and John Dodson found a relationship between stress and performance.
      1. To a certain point, a specific amount of stress is healthy, useful, and even beneficial.
         a) Not only to performance but also to one's health and well-being.
         b) The **Yerkes-Dodson Principle** explains that to a point, stress or arousal can increase performance.
            (1) To a point, as stress levels increase, so does performance.
            (2) When stress exceeds one's ability to cope, this overload contributes to diminished performance, inefficiency, and even health problems.
      2. Picture stress as a guitar string.
         a) Strung too tightly (too much tension), it will sound a note higher than is desirable.
            (1) When tightened to its maximum it is likely to snap.
         b) If not tightened sufficiently, it will play a note that is lower than is desirable.
            (1) If it is strung without any tension, no sound will come from it at all.
         c) The right amount of tension results in a perfectly and desirably sounding note.
            (1) The same image can be used to depict the healthiness of one's body with too much or too little stress.

IV. **THE TERMINOLOGY OF STRESS**
  A. Good and Bad Stress
    1. A **stressor** is any event or situation that is perceived by an individual as a threat which causes him or her to either adapt or initiate the stress response.
      a) A stressor is a stimulus and stress is a response.
      b) The stressor is the cause and stress is the effect.
    2. **Eustress,** a term coined by Dr. Hans Selye coined the term is the positive, desirable stress that keeps life interesting and helps to motivate and inspire.
      a) Going off to college, getting married, starting a new job, or having a baby can be happy, joyous, *and* stress-producing occasions.
      b) Eustress implies that a certain amount of stress is useful, beneficial and even good for our health, much like the perfectly strung guitar string.
    3. **Distress** refers to the negative effects of stress that drain us of energy and surpass our capacities to cope.
      a) Distress occurs when stress continues to increase, yet performance begins to decline. See Figure 1.2
  B. Acute and Chronic Stress
    1. **Acute stress** is the result of short-term stressors.
      a) Examples:
        (1) While out for a leisurely evening stroll a large, mangy dog leaps from the bushes, growling, with teeth bared.
        (2) While cruising down the highway, relaxing to your favorite tunes, a glance in your rearview mirror shows the flashing lights of a police car bearing down from behind.
    2. **Episodic acute stress** describes people who experience frequent episodes of acute stress.
      a) This is the person who elicits the response "What now?" when you see them racing toward you.
      b) It seems they are always in a rush, but usually late.
      c) If something can go wrong, it will.
      d) They often blame their problems on other people and external events.
      e) People experiencing these frequent episodes of acute stress tend to be over-aroused, short-tempered, irritable, anxious, and tense.
      f) They may describe themselves as having "a lot of nervous energy."
    3. **Chronic stress** results from the unrelenting demands and pressures that go on for interminable periods of time.
      a) The effects of chronic stress are fatigue, poor health and many other problems (See boxed off item called "Put the Glass Down.")
      b) This is the grinding stress that can wear you down day after day, year after year.
V. **HOLISTIC HEALTH**
  A. It is important to understand the relationship between health and stress.
    1. Here are two important points about health:
      a) Health is more than just the absence of disease.
        (1) Holistic health focuses on increasing your capacities for dealing with stress so you can enjoy optimal health and well-being.
      b) Health is more than just physical. (See Figure 1.3)
        (1) **Holistic health** includes the physical, intellectual, emotional, spiritual and social dimensions.
        (2) Imbalance in any of these dimensions will affect your health.
    2. The holistically healthy person functions as a total, balanced person.
VI. **DIMENSIONS OF HEALTH** (See figure 1.3)
  A. Physical Health
    1. When the cells, tissues, organs, and systems that function together to form your body are in good working order, you experience **physical health**.

2. Taking care of your body through healthy nutrition and exercise, adequate sleep, avoidance of alcohol and drug abuse, and regular health screenings are examples of promotion of health in the physical dimension.
3. Stress is a risk factor for many of the serious health problems that plague our society today.
4. Stress can cause disease and illness and disease and illness can cause stress.

B. Intellectual Health
1. **Intellectual health**, also called mental health, relates to your ability to think and learn from experiences, your ability to assess and question new information, and your openness to new learning.
2. Learning about stress is an important first step in preventing and managing stress.

C. Emotional Health
1. **Emotional health** pertains to feelings.
    a) It involves experiencing and appreciating a wide range of feelings and an ability to express these feelings and emotions in a healthy manner.
    b) The emotionally healthy individual uses healthy coping skills to keep from becoming overwhelmed by feelings of anger, fear, worry, love, guilt, or loneliness.
    c) Dealing successfully with stress means you take control of your emotions, rather than your emotions taking control of you.

D. Spiritual Health
1. **Spiritual health** relates to the morals and values that guide you and that give meaning, direction, and purpose to your life.
    a) It refers to your conviction that your life is meaningful and a belief that your life is guided by a reality greater than yourself
    b) Spiritually healthy people believe their life has value and that they are here for a reason.
    c) Much of stress in today's society relates to being out of touch with our values and beliefs.

E. Social Health
1. **Social health** refers to the ability to relate to others and express care and concern for others.
2. The ability to interact effectively with others, to develop satisfying interpersonal relationships, and to fulfill social roles is important for social health.
3. When you are socially healthy, you feel accepted by others and see yourself as an important part of your world.
4. A strong social support system increases the capacity for handling the demands of life.
    a) People who have the support of friends and family are better able to deal with the ups and downs of life.

VII. HOLISTIC HEALTH: PUTTING IT ALL TOGETHER

A. Review the Holistic Stress Checklist (Table 1.1) to see how stress affects every dimension of health.
B. Everyone is unique. Many factors play a part in how people react to stressors.
1. Genetic variations may partly explain the differences in how we react to stressors.
2. Some people are just naturally laid-back, while others react strongly at the slightest hint of stress.
3. Life experiences may also increase your sensitivity to stress.
4. Strong stress reactions sometimes can be traced to early environmental factors.
5. People who were exposed to extreme stress as children tend to be particularly vulnerable to stress as adults.

VIII. SOURCES OF STRESS

A. Some common stressors that relate to many college students. (See Figure 1.4 Top 10 Impediments to Academic Performance)
1. Time Management
2. Personal Expectations
3. Family Expectations and Family Life
4. Employment Decisions and Finances

    5. School Pressures
    6. Living Arrangements
    7. Relationships
    8. Physical Health Issues
    9. Environmental Stressors
    10. Information Overload
    11. Choices
    12. Daily Hassles

IX. CONCLUSION

   A. In *Stress Management for Life* you will learn that stress can be prevented and managed through three basic approaches. You can:
1. Eliminate the stressor - By confronting the problems causing you stress, you can sometimes change or eliminate the source of the stress.
2. Change your thinking - There are times when the cause of your stress can not be eliminated, but you always have the power to change your interpretation of the situation and the way you think about it.
3. Manage the stress - Sometimes the best we can do is manage the stress through skills that help us cope most successfully. Relaxation techniques help you manage the effects of stress.

   B. Using the tools of this book you will learn:
1. The factors causing negative stress for you.
2. How stress affects you physically, emotionally, mentally, spiritually, and socially.
3. How to increase your *capacity* for handling the demands that are part of today's world.
4. How to prevent stress.
5. How to manage and cope successfully with the stress you can't prevent.

LEARNING ACTIVITIES

ACTIVITY 1 - JOURNALING

Objective: The purpose of this activity is to encourage critical thinking and honest personal reflection on topics relating to the chapter content. Explore personal thoughts, feelings, values, and behaviors as you selectively incorporate stress management knowledge and behaviors into your plan for improved health through better stress management.

Instructions: You will find journaling questions in each chapter of your Activities Manual. These questions relate specifically to the chapter content. Moving your thoughts from your mind to the paper is a powerful strategy for relieving stress and for increasing awareness of your thoughts, feelings and behaviors. Your course instructor can provide further guidance on how to complete this activity.

Complete the following journaling questions. Select the questions that have the most relevance for you.

1. What is your own personal definition of stress? What does stress mean to you?
2. How do you think you are doing in each of the five dimensions of health? Give examples from your personal experience. The dimension of health that I probably need to work on the most is …
3. Finish this sentence with your own thoughts: My feelings about my current state of health are …
4. Do you agree that the spiritual dimension of health is the foundation for health? If so, why? If not, what dimension do you believe is the most important? Why?
5. According to the FYI survey results, college women feel overwhelmed more frequently than college men. Why do you think this is probably the case?
6. What do you see are the main stressors for you as a college student? How you think yours compare with other students?
7. How does the information in this chapter affect you personally? What insights did you have about yourself and the stress that you experience?
8. Respond to the following statement: I think that the stressors that I currently experience have most to do with my heredity, my environment, or my life experiences or some combination of these. I feel that way because …

ACTIVITY 2 - HOW BALANCED ARE YOU?

Objective: The purpose of this activity is to provide you with an opportunity to assess your personal level of balance in each dimension of health.

Instructions: Using a piece of paper or index card, draw your body representing how balanced you think you are in each of the dimensions of health using the following directions:
- Head represents the intellectual dimension
- Trunk represents the spiritual dimension
- One arm represents emotional dimension
- Other arm represents social dimension
- One leg represents physical dimension
- Other leg represents occupational/work dimension (this would include school)

If you feel balanced and satisfied with the time and energy spent on your intellectual dimension, for example, your head will appear proportional to the rest of their body. If you think you spend too much time and energy on this dimension, your head will be large; not enough and your head would be small in proportion to the rest of the body. If you are not taking time for the physical dimension (exercise, sleep, nutrition), your leg may appear very small. If you are doing nothing for spiritual health, your trunk will be disproportionately small. A "normal", proportional body will indicate balance in all dimensions.

5

ACTIVITY 3- CLARIFYING DIMENSIONS

Objective: The purpose of this activity is to help you expand your understanding of each of the 5 dimensions of health.

Instructions: Think through each of the dimensions of health as outlined in the text. Brainstorm answers to the following discussion items:
1. Define or describe the components of the dimension
2. Tell what it means to function optimally in the dimension - what would be characteristics of a healthy person in this dimension?
3. What are some ways that a person can improve or enhance the functioning of this dimension?
4. What can go wrong in this dimension - what health concerns may arise in the dimension?
5. In what ways does adverse or positive functioning of the dimension negatively or positively affect the other dimensions?

<u>**RELATED WEBSITES**</u>

The Mind-Body Medical Institute

Resource page to the Harvard Mind/Body Clinic. Extensive Information.

http://www.mbmi.org/

HealthWorld Online

Provides 10 categories of health and wellness topics for consumers and professionals including nutrition, mind-body connection, and a medical library.

http://www.healthy.net/

Healthopedia

A medical and health consumer information resource containing comprehensive and unbiased information in patient-friendly language from trusted sources on over 1,500 health topics, 70 focused health centers, and more than 11,000 drugs and medications.

http://www.healthopedia.com/

CHAPTER 2
SELF-ASSESSMENT

<u>CHAPTER OUTLINE</u>
Use this outline to take notes as you read the chapter in the text and/or as your instructor lectures in class.

I. **SELF-ASSESSMENT**
    A. One of the looming challenges for successful stress management is to determine what causes you stress.
        1. A certain level of stress can energize and motivate you to deal with the important issues in your life.
        2. You will want to focus your energy on the things in your life that are truly important. How do you determine what factors cause you unnecessary stress? How does your stress level compare to others?
    B. A variety of assessments will help you answer these questions.

II. **WHERE ARE YOU NOW STRESS-WISE?**
    A. The first step in developing a plan to help you manage your stress is assessment.
    B. In this chapter, you will find a variety of tools to help assess your stress levels.
    C. The information you gain from the assessments in this chapter should be used as it seems relevant to you and your life.
    D. These assessments and surveys are not intended to be diagnostic, but only to guide you in better understanding yourself.

III. **ASSESS YOUR STRESS**
    A. The first self-assessment is the Assess Your Stress activity. See Figure 2.1. It includes the following:
        1. Resting Heart Rate
            a) After you have been sitting or relaxing for a period of time, find your pulse.
                (1) Your **radial pulse** can be found on the thumb side of your wrist.
                (2) Your **carotid pulse** can be found on your neck just under the jaw.
            b) Count the number of beats for sixty seconds.
            c) Place this number in the Assess Stress Table.
        2. Breathing pattern
            a) Sit in a chair so your back is primarily straight up and down against the backrest.
            b) Place one hand on your abdomen with your palm covering your navel.
            c) While sitting straight up, notice your breath as it goes in and comes back out.
                (1) Notice which hand moves more - your chest or your abdominal hand.
            d) In the Assess Stress Table choose the way you are breathing - abdomen, chest, or both.
        3. Respiration Rate
            a) While sitting, breathe normally and naturally.
                (1) Count how many natural, effortless breaths you take in a minute. This is called **respiration rate.**
                (2) Each inhalation and exhalation cycle is considered one breath.
            b) Record the number of breaths you take per minute in the Assess Your Stress table.
        4. Stress-o-meter
            a) Think back over the waking hours of the last month of your life. Give yourself a rating according to the following scale.
                (1) A score of "1" would indicate that you feel your life has been relatively stress-free during that period. You have felt blissful and calm at all times. Everything seemed to go your way. A "10" score would mean that you felt extremely anxious most of the time and

that this was a month packed with high levels of stress. You felt totally overwhelmed, like your life was out of control, and like you were unable to cope.
    (2) If you were to average out the month (we all have highs and lows), what number would you give yourself on this scale from 1 to 10?
    (3) Record this number on the Assess Your Stress Table.
- B. Assess Your Stress Results - How you scored each of these simple measures may be indicative of higher stress levels. Each of these might indicate high stress:
    1. Higher resting heart rates
        a) Normal heart rates range between 70 and 80 beats per minute.
    2. Chest breathing
        a) Chest breathing indicates activation of the fight or flight response.
    3. High breathing Rate
        a) The average respiration rate is 12-16 breaths per minute.
        b) A faster breathing rate might be an indicator of higher-than-desired stress levels.
    4. High perceived stress levels
        a) May indicate continued activation of the stress response.

IV. SYMPTOMS OF STRESS ASSESSMENT
- A. The symptoms of stress table (Figure 2.2) gives students another look at how and to what extent common symptoms of chronic stress may be affecting them.
    1. The more often you experience these symptoms of stress, the more likely it is that stress is having a negative impact on your life.

V. PERCEIVED STRESS SCALE (PSS)
- A. The PSS is a classic stress assessment instrument. See Figure 2.3.
    1. The questions in this scale ask about your feelings and thoughts during the last month.
    2. The best approach is to answer each question fairly quickly.
    3. Individual scores on the PSS can range from 0 to 40 with higher scores indicating higher perceived stress.
    4. The Perceived Stress Scale is interesting and important because your perception of what is happening in your life is your most important determinant of how you are doing.

VI. THE INVENTORY OF COLLEGE STUDENTS' RECENT LIFE EXPERIENCES (ICSRLE)
- A. The ICSRLE was designed to identify individual exposure to sources of stress or hassles. See Figure 2.4.
- B. This inventory also allows for an identification of the extent to which those stressors were experienced over the past month.
- C. The ICSRLE was developed uniquely for college students.
- D. Your score on the ICSRLE can range from 0 to 147.
    1. Higher scores indicate higher levels of exposure to hassles.
        a) You can determine your current level of stress by adding your score for each hassle.
        b) You can discover which hassles play a greater part in your life by observing those items for which you scored a 3.

VII. THE ARDELL WELLNESS STRESS TEST
- A. The Ardell Wellness Stress Test incorporates physical, mental, emotional, spiritual, and social aspects of health for a balanced assessment. See Figure 2.5.
    1. This assessment is based on your personal perception of satisfaction about various aspects of your life.
        a) A higher overall score indicates less stress and overall well-being.
        b) A lower overall score indicates an increased need for doing something about your stress levels.

VIII. STUDENT STRESS SCALE
- A. The Student Stress Scale is an adaptation for college students of the Life Events Scale developed by Holmes and Rahe. See Figure 2.6.

B. It was designed to predict the likelihood of disease and illness following exposure to stressful life events.
  1. Higher scores indicate increased exposure to potential stressors
     a) Each life event is given a score that indicates the amount of readjustment a person has to make as a result of change.
     b) Higher scores have been found to correlate with higher likelihood of suffering from common symptoms of stress - such as getting sick in the near future.
C. It is important to note that this assessment considers only the events that occur, not individual perception of these events in life.

IX. TOMBSTONE TEST
A. When all is said and done, one of the most important assessments may be the Tombstone Test. How do you want to be remembered?
  1. Do you want to be remembered for being a workaholic?
  2. Do you want to be remembered as the one who always won the argument?
  3. Do you want to be remembered for making more money than your neighbor?
  4. Do you want to be remembered as the one who never forgave someone who wronged you?
  5. Do you want to be remembered as a good parent, spouse, and friend?
  6. Do you want to be remembered as someone who was whole and balanced in body, mind, and spirit?
  7. Do you want to be remembered for the service you provided to those who needed help?
     a) Make a list of these qualities for which you would like to be remembered.
     b) Ask yourself, are you living your life in a way that demonstrates the qualities you value?
  8. When your choices are guided by the values and goals that are most important to you, your life can be full and active, yet not stressful.
  9. Decide how you want to be remembered - and then live your life to that effect.

X. DAILY STRESS DIARY
A. The purpose of a food diary is to record everything you eat to increase your awareness of what you are eating.
B. The Daily Stress Log serves the same purpose, only relating to your stress
  1. For several days, you will make a note of any and all activities that put a strain on energy and time, trigger anger or anxiety, or precipitate a negative physical response.
  2. When you have completed a daily log for a few days, review the log and identify 2 or 3 stressful events or activities that you can modify or eliminate.
  3. As you keep track of all of the events that happen during a day, and you notice patterns in which you find yourself getting more stressed, you can begin to take steps to make adjustments in those damaging patterns.

XI. CONCLUSION
A. In this chapter you have had the opportunity to assess your stress from many different perspectives:
  1. Looking back over each of the assessment surveys and tools you will see that these tools measured stress from a variety of perspectives including:
     a) Physiological indicators of stress.
     b) Your perception of what is happening in your life.
     c) Sources of stress and frequency of hassles.
     d) Your level of satisfaction with events in your life.
     e) Type of life events you have experienced.

<u>LEARNING ACTIVITIES</u>

ACTIVITY 1 - JOURNALING

Objective: The purpose of this activity is to encourage critical thinking and honest personal reflection on topics relating to the chapter content. Explore personal thoughts, feelings, values, and behaviors as you selectively incorporate stress management knowledge and behaviors into your plan for improved health through better stress management.

Instructions: You will find journaling questions in each chapter of your Activities Manual. These questions relate specifically to the chapter content. Moving your thoughts from your mind to the paper is a powerful strategy for relieving stress and for increasing awareness of your thoughts, feelings and behaviors. Your course instructor can provide further guidance on how to complete this activity.

Complete the following journaling questions. Select the questions that have the most relevance for you.

1. What are your thoughts about the results of your stress assessments? Did any of the results surprise you? Did you disagree with any of your results?
2. Respond to this statement: My feelings about my current levels of stress are …
3. Respond to this statement: If I could change one thing about my stress, it would be…
4. What are the main things that really make you feel stress?
5. You can understand after reading this chapter that assessing stress is not a simple matter. What other factors might be included to assess and understand your stress?
6. Have you lived abroad or traveled to other countries? If so, what have you observed about stress in other cultures? Do you think the U.S. is a "high-stress" culture related to others you have experienced? Is this the inevitable price we pay for high productivity?
7. How does the information in this chapter affect you personally? What insights did you have about yourself and the stress that you experience?

ACTIVITY 2 - STRESS SELF-ASSESSMENT

Objectives: The purpose of this activity is to help you get a sense of your current stress level through a variety of self-assessment instruments.

Materials needed:
- Handout 2:1 Assess Your Stress and Symptoms of Stress Form
- Handout 2:2 Perceived Stress Scale (PSS)
- Handout 2:3 The Inventory of College Students' Recent Life Experiences
- Handout 2:4 The Ardell Wellness Stress Test
- Handout 2:5 Student Stress Scale

Duration of Activity: 25-30 minutes

Description of Activity: Complete each of the self-assessments listed above. These handouts are found later in this chapter and also in chapter 2 of the text. Follow the instructions included with each self-assessment.

ACTIVITY 3 - DAILY STRESS DIARY

Objective: The purpose of this activity is to record feelings of stress as it happens to increase your awareness of situations and ways of thinking that tend to promote stress.

Instructions:
1. Complete Handout 2.6 Daily Stress Diary for at least 2-3 days, including at least 1 weekend day. You will need to make additional copies of the diary for each day.

2. Make a note of any and all activities that put a strain on your energy and time, trigger anger or anxiety, or precipitate a negative physical response. Also note reactions to these stressful events.
3. When you have completed the diary for a few days, review the diary and identify 2 or 3 stressful events or activities that you can modify or eliminate.

ACTIVITY 4 - STRESS ASSESS INTERNET ACTIVITY

You might prefer an online option for assessing stress. The University of Wisconsin - Stevens Point (UWSP) has long been a leader in the area of health and wellness. UWSP Health Service offers three valuable online stress assessments. To access the site, go to the website below:
http://wellness.uwsp.edu/Other/stress/
You will have the option of choosing three different assessments; Stress Sources, Distress Symptoms, and Stress Balancing Strategies. Each provides individualized assessment information that can help you grow in your understanding of stress in your life.

HANDOUTS
2.1 Assess Your Stress and Symptoms of Stress
2.2 Perceived Stress Scale
2.3 The Inventory of College Students' Recent Life Experiences
2.4 The Ardell Wellness Stress Test
2.5 Student Stress Scale
2.6 Daily Stress Diary

Handout 2.1 Assess Your Stress and Symptoms of Stress

Assess Your Stress

Resting Heart Rate	_____ Beats per minute
Breathing Pattern	_____ Abdomen _____ Chest _____ Both
Respiration Rate	_____ Breaths per minute
Stress-o-meter	1 2 3 4 5 6 7 8 9 10

Symptoms of Stress

Symptoms	Frequency of symptoms						
	Almost all day, every day	Once or twice daily	Every night or day	2-3 times per week	Once a week	Once a month	Never
Headaches							
Tense muscles, sore neck and back							
Fatigue							
Anxiety, worry, phobias							
Difficulty falling asleep							
Insomnia							
Bouts of anger/hostility							
Boredom, depression							
Eating too much or too little							
Diarrhea, cramps, gas, constipation							
Tics, restlessness, itching							

Handout 2.2 Perceived Stress Scale (PSS)

For each question choose from the following alternatives:

0 - Never

1 - Almost never

2 - Sometimes

3 - Fairly often

4 - Very often

_____1.   In the last month, how often have you been upset because of something that happened unexpectedly?

_____2.   In the last month, how often have you felt that you were unable to control the important things in your life?

_____3.   In the last month, how often have you felt nervous and "stressed"?

_____4.   In the last month, how often have you felt confident about your ability to handle your personal problems?

_____5.   In the last month, how often have you felt that things were going your way?

_____6.   In the last month, how often have you found that you could not cope with all the things that you had to do?

_____7.   In the last month, how often have you been able to control irritations in your life?

_____8.   In the last month, how often have you felt that you were on top of things?

_____9.   In the last month, how often have you been angered because of things that happened that were outside of your control?

_____10. In the last month, how often have you felt difficulties were piling up so high that you could not overcome them?

Figuring your PSS score:

You can determine your PSS score by following these directions:

First, reverse your scores for questions 4, 5, 7, and 8. On these 4 questions, change the scores like this: 0 = 4, 1 = 3, 2 = 2, 3 = 1, and 4 = 0. For all other questions, use the number you wrote down as the score.

Now add up your scores for each item to get a total. **My total score is _____.**

*Scores ranging from 0-13 would be considered **low perceived stress**.*

*Scores ranging from 14-26 would be considered **moderate perceived stress**.*

*Scores ranging from 27-40 would be considered **high perceived stress**.*

Handout 2.3 Inventory of College Students' Recent Life Experiences (ICSRLE)

The following is a list of experiences that many students have at some time or other. Indicate for each experience how much it has been a part of your life over the past month. Mark your answers according to the following guide:

Intensity of Experience over the Past Month

0 = not at all part of my life

1 = only slightly part of my life

2 = distinctly part of my life

3 = very much part of my life

_____1. Conflicts with boyfriend's/girlfriend's/spouse's family

_____2. Being let down or disappointed by friends

_____3. Conflict with professor(s)

_____4. Social rejection

_____5. Too many things to do at once

_____6. Being taken for granted

_____7. Financial conflicts with family members

_____8. Having your trust betrayed by a friend

_____9. Separation from people you care about

_____10. Having your contributions overlooked

_____11. Struggling to meet your own academic standards

_____12. Being taken advantage of

_____13. Not enough leisure time

_____14. Struggling to meet the academic standards of others

_____15. A lot of responsibilities

_____16. Dissatisfaction with school

_____17. Decisions about intimate relationship(s)

_____18. Not enough time to meet your obligations

_____19. Dissatisfaction with your mathematical ability

_____20. Important decisions about your future career

_____21. Financial burdens

_____22. Dissatisfaction with your reading ability

_____23. Important decisions about your education

_____24. Loneliness

_____25. Lower grades than you hoped for

_____26. Conflict with teaching assistant(s)

_____27. Not enough time for sleep

_____28. Conflicts with your family

_____29. Heavy demands from extracurricular activities

_____30. Finding courses too demanding

_____31. Conflicts with friends

_____32. Hard effort to get ahead

_____33. Poor health of a friend

_____34. Disliking your studies

_____35. Getting "ripped off" or cheated in the purchase of services

_____36. Social conflicts over smoking

_____37. Difficulties with transportation

_____38. Disliking fellow student(s)

_____39. Conflicts with boyfriend/girlfriend/spouse

_____40. Dissatisfaction with your ability at written expression

_____41. Interruptions of your school work

_____42. Social isolation

_____43. Long waits to get service (at banks, stores, etc.)

_____44. Being ignored

_____45. Dissatisfaction with your physical appearance

_____46. Finding course(s) uninteresting

_____47. Gossip concerning someone you care about

_____48. Failing to get expected job

_____49. Dissatisfaction with your athletic skills

Scoring the ICSRLE

Add your total points: _____

Your score on the ICSRLE can range from 0 to 147. Higher scores indicate higher levels of exposure to hassles. From your results, focus on two key outcomes:

1. Determine your current level of stress by adding your score for each hassle and getting a total.

2. Discover which hassles play a greater part in your life. Items that you rated "3" indicate that those stressors are more of an issue for you.

Handout 2.4 Ardell Wellness Stress Test

This assessment is based on your personal perception of satisfaction. Rate your satisfaction with each of the following items by using this scale:

+ 3 = Ecstatic   -1 = Mildly disappointed

+ 2 = Very happy   - 2 = Very disappointed

+ 1 = Mildly happy   - 3 = Completely dismayed

 0 = Indifferent

_____ 1.   Choice of career (or major)

_____ 2.   Present job/ business/ school

_____ 3.   Marital status

_____ 4.   Primary relationships

_____ 5.   Capacity to have fun

_____ 6.   Amount of fun experienced in last month

_____ 7.   Financial prospects

_____ 8.   Current income level

_____ 9.   Spirituality

_____ 10.   Level of self-esteem

_____ 11.   Prospects for having impact on those who know you and possibly others

_____ 12.   Sex life

_____ 13.   Body—how it looks and performs

_____ 14.   Home life

_____ 15.   Life skills and knowledge of issues and facts unrelated to your job or profession

_____ 16.   Learned stress management capacities

_____ 17.   Nutritional knowledge, attitudes, and choices

_____ 18.   Ability to recover from disappointment, hurts, setbacks, and tragedies

_____ 19.   Confidence that you currently are, or will be in the future, reasonably close to your highest potential

_____ 20.   Achievement of a rounded or balanced quality in your life

_____ 21.   Sense that life for you is on an upward curve, getting better and fuller all the time

_____ 22.   Level of participation in issues and concerns beyond your immediate interests

_____ 23.   Choice whether to parent or not, and with the consequences or results of that choice

_____ 24.   Role in some kind of network of friends, relatives, and/or others about whom you care deeply and who reciprocate that commitment to you

_____ 25.   Emotional acceptance of the inescapable reality of aging

Total _____

(Ardell Wellness Stress Test continued on next page)

Ardell Wellness Stress Test Interpretation

+51 to +75 You are a self-actualized person, nearly immune from the ravages of stress. There are few, if any, challenges likely to distract you from a sense of near total well-being.

+25 to +50 You have mastered the wellness approach to life and have the capacity to deal creatively and efficiently with events and circumstances.

+1 to +24 You are a wellness-oriented person, with an ability to prosper as a whole person, but you should give a bit more attention to optimal health concepts and skill building.

0 to -24 You are a candidate for additional training in how to deal with stress. A sudden increase in potentially negative events and circumstances could cause a severe emotional setback.

-25 to -50 You are a candidate for counseling. You are either too pessimistic or have severe problems in dealing with stress.

-51 to -75 You are a candidate for major psychological care with virtually no capacity for coping with life's problems.

Handout 2.5 Student Stress Scale

For each event that occurred in your life within the past year, record the corresponding score. If an event occurred more than once, multiply the score for that event by the number of times the event occurred and record that score. Total all the scores.

Life Event	Value	Your Score
1. Death of a close family member	100	
2. Death of a close friend	73	
3. Divorce of parents	65	
4. Jail term	63	
5. Major personal injury or illness	63	
6. Marriage	58	
7. Getting fired from a job	50	
8. Failing an important course	47	
9. Change in the health of a family member	45	
10. Pregnancy	45	
11. Sex problems	44	
12. Serious argument with a close friend	40	
13. Change in financial status	39	
14. Change of academic major	39	
15. Trouble with parents	39	
16. New girlfriend or boyfriend	37	
17. Increase in workload at school	37	
18. Outstanding personal achievement	36	
19. First semester/quarter in college	36	
20. Change in living conditions	31	
21. Serious argument with an instructor	30	
22. Getting lower grades than expected	29	
23. Change in sleeping habits	29	
24. Change in social activities	29	
25. Change in eating habits	28	
26. Chronic car trouble	26	
27. Change in number of family get-togethers	26	
28. Too many missed classes	25	
29. Changing colleges	24	
30. Dropping more than one class	23	
31. Minor traffic violations	20	
	Your Total Score	

Score Interpretation:

Researchers determined that if your total score is:

300 or more — statistically you stand an almost 80 percent chance of getting sick in the near future.

150 to 299 — you have a 50-50 chance of experiencing a serious health change within two years.

149 or less — you have about a 30 percent chance of a serious health change.[*]

Handout 2.6 Daily Stress Diary

Name: _____   Date: _____

Time	Place	Situation initiating the stress response (source of stress)	Level of Perceived Stress*	Thoughts and feelings about the stressor including coping strategies

*Perceived Stress level: 1 = Slight   2 = Moderate 3 = Strong   4 = Intense

Major sources of stress today:

Assessment of how you managed stress today:

RELATED WEBSITES:

Discovering Your Stress Type

Are you a Drifter, a Speed Freak, or perhaps a Loner when it comes to handling stress? Take this survey to find out.

http://stress.about.com/cs/inthenews/a/ucstresstypes.htm

Self Assessment Index

Each assessment is FREE and is designed to help you find more out about yourself and how you can improve your health.

http://www.internethealthlibrary.com/sq/self-assess-list.htm

StressCare Sress Self Assessment

Another Stress Self Assessment by StressCare

http://www.stresscare.com/global/index.html

CHAPTER 3
THE SCIENCE OF STRESS

CHAPTER OUTLINE
Use this outline to take notes as you read the chapter in the text and/or as your instructor lectures in class.

I.   **STRESS AND THE BIG BEAR**
   A.   Why do you feel stress in the first place?
   B.   To answer these questions, we need to go back a few thousand years to see what life was like back then. This will help us understand how our bodies are programmed to respond to threats and danger today.
   C.   Imagine a scenario in which we are having a barbeque many thousand years ago. As we are enjoying each other's company, a big bear emerges from a nearby forest. Our first thought sound something like "Uh-Oh, I'm in danger" followed closely by the thought to either run for safety or fight this bear to protect ourselves and our friends. We call this automatic immediate reaction to the thought that we are in danger the fight-or-flight response.

II. **FIGHT-OR-FLIGHT RESPONSE**
   A.   A flood of physiological processes in the body takes place automatically, immediately and precisely after the initial awareness of danger.
   B.   Harvard physiologist Walter Cannon coined the term **fight-or-flight response** to describe our body's automatic response when we perceive threat or danger
   C.   This is a primitive response that gives us strength, power, and speed to avoid physical harm.
   D.   The fight-or-flight response is designed to help us do one thing, and only one thing, very well: SURVIVE.
      1.   Whether the response culminates in "fight" or "flight" depends on whether the threat or stressor is perceived as surmountable.
   E.   Figure 3.1 shows the sequence of events in the fight-or-flight response
      1.   **Homeostasis** is when the body functions efficiently and comfortably.
      2.   Then something happens in our environment - anything that is the equivalent of a big bear charging out of the forest.
      3.   This perception of danger automatically initiates the fight-or-flight response.
      4.   Once we sense no more danger, we experience exhaustion and fatigue because we have expended a tremendous amount of energy while running or fighting.
         a)   We are exhausted but the stress response is no longer activated. Because we feel safe again, the functions in the body that activate the stress response are turned off, and we gradually return to normal (homeostasis).

III. **PHYSIOLOGICAL RESPONSE TO STRESS**
   A.   When the stress response is initiated, immediate and powerful changes come about because of the activation of the nervous system called the **autonomic nervous system** (ANS).
      1.   The ANS is responsible for many functions in the body that occur involuntarily such as digestion, heart rate, blood pressure, and body temperature.
      2.   The activity of the autonomic nervous system takes place completely beyond our conscious control. It is automatic.
   B.   There are two branches of the ANS that are designed to regulate the fight-or-flight response.
      1.   The **sympathetic nervous system** (SNS) is the part of the ANS responsible for initiating the fight-or-flight response, each time we have a thought of potential danger or pain.
         a)   We only need to think that we are in danger and the flood of physiological and emotional activity is turned on to increase power, speed, and strength.
      2.   The **parasympathetic nervous system** (PNS) is the branch of nervous system activity designed to return the physiology to a state of homeostasis, or balance, after the threat, danger, or potential pain is no longer perceived to be imminent.
         a)   Responsible for counterbalancing the sympathetic activity that restores

calm, promotes relaxation, and facilitates digestive functions, energy storage, and tissue repair and growth.

C. The ANS is controlled by the **hypothalamus** located in the central portion of the brains.
   1. Plays a key role in the stress response because it is the chief region for integration of sympathetic and parasympathetic activities.
   2. When the hypothalamus receives the message of danger from the higher-order thinking part of the mind it is like an alarm system going off. The message is swiftly delivered through the nervous system to every other system of the body.
   3. The hypothalamus also delivers a message to the endocrine system to initiate the secretion of stress hormones.
      a) Adrenalin (**epinephrine** and **norepinephrine**) are produced by the adrenal glands.
      b) **Cortisol** is released from a portion of the adrenal glands called the **adrenal cortex**.
      c) These hormones flood every cell in the body with the specific message to prepare for fight-or-flight, for more power and speed when we are faced with an imminent threat.

D. Autonomic Nervous System Responses (See Figure 3.2 Effects of Stress on the Body)
   1. Immediate physiological changes that result from sympathetic nervous system activation.
   2. Nervous system processes in the body that decrease in functioning when the fight-or-flight response is activated.
      a) We do not need this last set of functions and systems to operate at high capacity to escape from threatening situations. Their work is therefore suppressed in order to divert energy to those vital systems involved in increasing speed and power.
   3. Understanding the nervous systems response to stress is important in explaining the stress-related diseases and conditions covered in the next chapter.

IV. **THE STRESS RESPONSE IN TODAY'S WORLD**
   A. In our current society, our bodies still react the same way to threats - real or imagined - even though, in a vast majority of cases, the stressor does not require us to fight or flee.
      1. The fight-or-flight emergency response is inappropriate to today's social stresses.
      2. Our ancestors survived by running away from or fighting their predators
         a) Today we have traffic jams and deadlines, loneliness and lack of money; different types of stressors, which do not include the need to run or fight.
         b) Our fight-or-flight response is an outdated mechanism that our primitive systems have not yet adapted to.
   B. Acute Stress
      1. In the short run, the stress response is very beneficial to help us amass great strength, focus more clearly, increase our speed, and perform at a higher level when a threat is present.
         a) We can occasionally use this immediate energy to help us when we find ourselves in actual danger, facing potential pain or even death.
      2. For most of us our society today is not one where *real* acute threat or danger is a daily occurrence.
   C. Chronic Stress (See Figure 3.3)
      1. Our body gives us feedback about unhealthy chronic stress with a host of signals indicating imbalance.
         a) Some of those signals, if not heeded, can even include damage to parts of the system.
         b) Although stress is not listed among the top 10 causes of death in America, it is linked to many illnesses.
            (1) This does not necessarily mean that stress causes the problem, but it does mean that stress contributes to the problem.

V. **THE GENERAL ADAPTATION SYNDROME**
    A. The process in which the body tries to adapt to chronic stress is known as the **general adaptation syndrome.**
    B. Stress pioneer Dr. Hans Selye researched the physiological effects of chronic stress on rats.
        1. He observed some specific responses whenever he injected an animal with a toxin.
        2. Earlier, as a medical student, he had noticed similar responses in people.
            a) Selye theorized that the same pattern of changes occurs in the body in reaction to any kind of stress and that the pattern is what eventually leads to disease conditions, such as ulcers, arthritis, hypertension, arteriosclerosis, or diabetes.
    C. See Figure 3.4 The Three Stages of Selye's General Adaptation Syndrome.
        1. Alarm Stage – When a stressor occurs, the body responds in the fight-or-flight response.
        2. Stage of Resistance - If the stressor continues, the body mobilizes its internal resources in an effort to return to a state of homeostasis, but because the perception of a threat still exists, complete homeostasis is not achieved.
            a) The stress response stays activated, usually at less intensity than during the alarm stage, but still at a level to cause hyperarousal.
        3. Stage of Exhaustion - If the stress continues long enough, the body can no longer function normally.
            a) Organ systems may fail and the body breaks down in a variety of ways.
            b) Continuous stress that causes the body to constantly adapt can become a threat to health.

VI. **THE STRESS RESPONSE AND YOU**
    A. Our fight-or-flight response is one example of the way that short bursts of heightened energy and vigilance can actually save our lives.
    B. But we aren't well adapted to deal with surges of adrenaline and cortisol day after day.

VII. **CONCLUSION**
    A. Your body is designed to respond to acute stress in a predictable manner for one outcome, your survival.
        1. The stress response is critical for your ability to survive the life-threatening situations in life.
        2. The physiological response is not well suited to deal with the common pressures and stressors of today.

LEARNING ACTIVITIES

ACTIVITY 1 - JOURNALING

Objective: The purpose of this activity is to encourage critical thinking and honest personal reflection on topics relating to the chapter content. Explore personal thoughts, feelings, values, and behaviors as you selectively incorporate stress management knowledge and behaviors into your plan for improved health through better stress management.

Instructions: You will find journaling questions in each chapter of your Activities Manual. These questions relate specifically to the chapter content. Moving your thoughts from your mind to the paper is a powerful strategy for relieving stress and for increasing awareness of your thoughts, feelings and behaviors. Your course instructor can provide further guidance on how to complete this activity.

Complete the following journaling questions. Select the questions that have the most relevance for you.

1. Explain in your own words how the fight-or-flight response works. How does this response contribute to your survival in life today?
2. Respond to the following statement: I noticed that these are the things that I feel and experience mentally, emotionally, and physically when I am stressed for a short period of time...
3. Respond to the following statement: I notice that these are the things that I feel and experience mentally, emotionally, and physically when I am stressed for a long period of time.
4. How does the information in this chapter affect you personally? What insights did you have about yourself and the stress that you experience?

ACTIVITY 2 - WHY STRESS

Objectives: The purpose of this discussion is to help you understand why you experience stress.

Description of Activity: Follow the information in chapter 3 using this scenario:
We are all together living in the wilds several thousand years ago. We are having a great time doing something fun like having a barbecue when a huge bear emerges from a nearby forest.
What is the first thought that you will have? Whatever it is, it will sound something like "Uh-oh!" "I'm in danger".
The next thought following "Uh-oh" will probably be "Run!" If there are people around who aren't able to run, you might also have the thought "Kill this bear so it doesn't hurt my family and friends!"
After that initial thought, a flood of physiological activity immediately happens throughout the body.

Write the words, "Fight or Flight" on the top of a piece of paper and underneath make a list of things that happen in the body during the fight or flight response. Use the information in Chapter 3 to help you create the list. Be sure to include normal functions which turn off during the fight-or-flight response, such as the immune system, the digestive system, and others listed in chapter 3.

Once the long list has been created ask yourself what you think the single purpose of all of this activity might be. The correct response is that the fight-or-flight response is designed for the single purpose of SURVIVAL. It has no other purpose.

Realize that the fight or flight response is designed to work for only a short period of time – Two to three minutes. By that time, our ancestors were either attacked by the bear or had fled for safety. Realize that fight-or-flight is an automatic response initiated by the autonomic nervous system. It happens automatically whenever we have any type of thought similar to "Uh-Oh!" We don't have to consciously get our heart rate pumping, increase the flood of adrenalin and cortisol, or increase our blood sugar. It all happens automatically. All we have to do is have the thought that we are in danger; we merely have to think of some threat we are about to encounter. The fight-or-flight response automatically kicks in.

ACTIVITY 3 - A REAL FIGHT-OR-FLIGHT SITUATION

Objectives: The purpose of this activity is to help you observe the powerful effects of the fight-or-flight response.

Description of Activity: Think back to a time in your life when you were in an actual situation where your life was really in danger. On a piece of paper, describe what was happening (perhaps you were being chased by someone or maybe you were in a house or building and you found out it was on fire and you had to escape quickly).

- Thoroughly describe the situation as it happened.
- Take a few moments to write down how you *felt* as this was happening. What flood of emotions did you notice yourself having?
- If you did need to run or use more power to deal with the situation, describe if you found yourself speedier or more powerful. What happened?
- Describe how you felt after the perilous situation had ended.
- Discuss how your experience was similar to the stress response as it is described in chapter 3 of your text.

ACTIVITY 4 - FIGHT-OR-FLIGHT OR TEND AND BEFRIEND

Objectives: The purpose of this activity is to invite you to distinguish differences in how men and women respond to stress.

Description of Activity: The tend-and-befriend theory states that women tend to respond to dangerous situations differently than men—women are more likely to do what is necessary to make sure those around them are safe and cared for whereas men follow the traditional course of the fight-or-flight— men are more likely to run from or fight the danger.

Explain why you either agree or disagree with the tend-and-befriend theory? In other words, do you think men and women have a different physiological response to stressors?

Think about situations you have seen where men and women were both in the same threatening situation. Did their responses to the threat support or oppose the tend-and-befriend theory?

RELATED WEBSITES

Discovery Health - Stress

Short article on the effects of stress on the body systems.

http://health.discovery.com/encyclopedias/illnesses.html?article=3096&page=1

teachhealth.com

Medical basis of stress, depression, anxiety, sleep problems, and drug use.

http://www.teachhealth.com/

About.com Stress management information site

Facts about stress

http://stress.about.com/cs/copingskills/a/stress101a.htm

CHAPTER 4
THE MIND/BODY CONNECTION

CHAPTER OUTLINE
Use this outline to take notes as you read the chapter in the text and/or as your instructor lectures in class.

I.   THE MIND/BODY CONNECTION
  A. What is going on with your mind and emotions is at least as, if not more important than what is happening in your body.
    1. In fact, what is going on in your mind determines what is happening in your body.
    2. Recently, researchers have been studying the mind-body connection to understand how thoughts and emotions relate to our experience with stress.

II. PSYCHOLOGICAL HEALTH
  A. Emotional health relates to feelings and the ability to achieve emotional balance.
  B. Mental health relates to a state in which the mind is engaged in lively, healthy interaction both internally and with the world around you
    1. Psychologically healthy people develop awareness and control of their thoughts and feelings.
      a) The outcome is a healthy and satisfying life.
      b) Individuals who are chronically pessimistic, angry, anxious or depressed are clearly more susceptible to stress and illness, including heart disease and cancer.
  C. What part does your mind play in your experience with stress?
    1. The stress response always starts with a thought.
    2. Scientific studies provide a solid foundation of undeniable scientific evidence explaining the connection between the body and the mind.

III. THE ROLE OF CHRONIC STRESS IN DISEASE
  A. Studies have shown that stress contributes to a significant percent of all major illnesses, including the number one cause of death in America, cardiovascular disease.
  B. Direct and indirect effects of chronic stress
    1. Direct effects of stress - physiological changes in the body.
      a) Hormones released by the endocrine system during the alarm reaction stage of the general adaptation syndrome affect the cardiovascular, immune, and other systems of the body.
    2. Indirect effects - unhealthy behaviors adopted by those with high stress levels.
      a) Individuals under more stress consume more alcohol, smoke more cigarettes, and drink more coffee than those under less stress.

IV. MEDIUM-TERM CHRONIC STRESS
  A. When we understand what is happening during the stress response, we can understand why medium-term effects of stress happen.
    1. Many functions in the body turn off because they are not needed to deal with danger.
    2. Other functions in the body are activated to higher than normal levels.
  B. Effects of Medium-Term Chronic Stress
    1. Muscle Tension and Pain
      a) When a muscle is told to fight or run for prolonged periods of time, it will remain in the contracted state longer than necessary.
        (1) When this happens, we notice two obvious results: pain and fatigue.
        (2) When a muscle stays contracted, it activates nervous system pain receptors that deliver the message of pain.
    2. Headaches
      a) If continually contracting muscles are on our head, the result is a headache.

      b) This explains why people take muscle relaxants to help them ease the pain of the headache.

3. Fatigue

      a) When a muscle is continually receiving the message to be ready for action, fatigue will result.

      b) It requires considerable energy for muscles to stay active.

4. Upset Stomach

      a) We do not need the digestive system for fight-or-flight situations.

      b) The digestive system ceases to effectively coordinate all of the processes necessary to break down food.

5. Difficulty sleeping

      a) It should not take more than a few minutes to fall asleep.

      b) We should also sleep comfortably through the entire night without waking up several times.

      c) If we are having a hard time falling asleep, it may be because our minds are thinking too much of other things.

         (1) Sleep-inducing brainwave activity can only happen as we are able to turn off the stress response.

      d) Insufficient sleep affects the immune system which leads to further health problems.

6. **Bruxism**

      a) Grinding, gnashing, or clenching your teeth during sleep or during situations that make you feel anxious or tense.

         (1) The third most common form of sleep disorder.

         (2) Psychological factors including anxiety, stress or tension, suppressed anger or frustration, or aggressive, competitive or hyperactive personality type are the causal factors.

7. Cold or sore throat

      a) During fight-or-flight the immune system is suppressed leading to increased likelihood of colds or flu.

C. Role of the Immune System

  1. Since the immune system is unable to work as effectively when you are stressed, you are more susceptible to every disease and illness that crosses your path.

D. The medium-term symptoms of chronic stress are the result of the stress response causing imbalances throughout normally functioning systems in the body.

  1. Whatever system turns on or off is in direct response to what we would need for flight-or-fight. When this happens for an extended period, health suffers.

V. LONG-TERM CHRONIC STRESS

A. While the medium-term effects of chronic stress are unpleasant and annoying, the long-term effects are dangerous and contribute to disease, suffering, and even death.

B. Stress and the heart

  1. Cardiovascular disease is the number one cause of death in the United States.

  2. Evidence suggests a relationship between the risk of cardiovascular disease and environmental and psychosocial factors.

  3. Acute and chronic stress may affect other risk factors for heart disease, such as high blood pressure and cholesterol levels, smoking, physical inactivity, and overeating.

      a) Mental stress increases oxygen demand because blood pressure and heart rate are elevated.

      b) Vascular resistance and coronary artery constriction during mental stress also decrease the blood supply. This results in decreased blood flow to the heart muscle.

      c) Blood tends to clot more easily. Your body is designed so you won't bleed to death. However, increased blood clotting in the blood vessels that surround the heart, or in the brain, can increase the chances that one of those clots may lodge itself on the wall of a blood vessel. If a clot is too big and the diameter of the blood vessel is too small, and if we add to that an increase in blood pressure which weakens the blood vessels, the result may be a heart attack or a stroke.

    d) Chronically high levels of cortisol may affect cardiac health by promoting inflammation that causes heart attacks.

C. Stress and the Immune System
    1. Stress suppresses the immune system's ability to produce and maintain **lymphocytes** (the white blood cells necessary for killing infection) and **natural killer cells** (the specialized cells that seek out and destroy foreign invaders), both crucial in the fight against disease and infection.
        a) Impaired immunity makes the body more susceptible to many diseases, including infections and disorders of the immune system itself such as the autoimmune disease rheumatoid arthritis.

D. Stress and Aging
    1. Chronic stress appears to accelerate the aging process by shortening the life span of cells, opening the door to disease.
        a) In one study, the cells of people under high stress aged the equivalent of 9 to 17 years more than the cells of people under little stress.
        b) In another study, caregivers who viewed their situation positively didn't seem to suffer the ill effects of stress as those who viewed their situation negatively.
        c) A common factor among people who live to be at least 100 years old is that they handle stress well.

E. Other disease conditions of stress
    1. Studies suggest that high levels of stress can trigger a large number of diseases and conditions - from obesity to ulcers.
        a) See text for a list of disease conditions associated with stress.

VI. **HOW THE MIND AND BODY COMMUNICATE**
A. An ever-increasing body of research documents the way in which attitudes, thoughts and emotions impact health.
    1. Sad or depressing thoughts produce changes in brain chemistry that have a detrimental affect on the body's physiology, and likewise, happy thoughts, loving thoughts of peace and tranquility, of compassion, friendliness, kindness, generosity, affection, warmth, and intimacy each produce a corresponding state of physiology via the flux of neurotransmitters and hormones in the central nervous system.

B. Psychosomatic Illness
    1. **Psychosomatic**, also called **psychophysiological**, conditions have both a mind and a body component.
    2. Candace Pert believes that "virtually all illness, if not psychosomatic in foundation, has a definite psychosomatic component. Recent technological innovations have allowed us to examine the molecular basis of the emotions, and to begin to understand how the molecules of our emotions share intimate connections with, and are indeed inseparable from, our physiology. It is the emotions, I have come to see, that link mind and body."
    3. Statistics show that single people and widows living alone are more likely to get cancer than people who are married.
        a) Their loneliness is called a risk factor - one could just as truly call it a carcinogen.

C. The Placebo and Nocebo Effect
    1. A phenomenon whereby an inactive substance or treatment is used to determine the effects of suggestion on the psychology, physiology, or biochemistry of experimental participants is known as the **placebo effect**.

2. In study after study, across a broad range of medical conditions, 25 to 35 percent of patients consistently experience satisfactory relief when placebos are used instead of regular medicines or procedures.
   a) The research supports the premise that belief that a treatment works does in fact result in increased effectiveness.
   b) One study suggested that the quality of the interaction between the patient and the physician can be extremely influential in patient outcomes and in some, perhaps many cases, patient and provider expectations and interactions may be more important than the specific treatments.
      (1) When the patient and the health care provider expect a treatment to be successful, the likelihood of success increases.
3. The causation of sickness and death by expectations of these negative outcomes and by associated emotional states is known as the **nocebo effect**.
   a) For example, when people who are susceptible to poison ivy are exposed to a harmless look-alike plant and told it is the real thing, they can develop a rash.
   b) In another study, cancer patients experienced hair loss when given a completely inert substance and told it was a powerful anticancer medicine that causes hair loss.

D. **Psychoneuroimmunology**
   1. A field of scientific inquiry that studies the chemical basis of communication between the body and mind as it relates to the nervous system and the immune system.
   2. The affects of a compromised immune system are far-reaching including everything from susceptibility to the common cold, to the rate of wound healing, and even a link with breast cancer development.
   3. A summary of studies demonstrate the effect of stress on the immune system.
      a) PNI research has shown that traumatic stress, such as the death of a loved one, can impair immunity for as long as a year.
      b) Studies of university students and staff in the United States and Spain have implicated stress and a generally negative outlook as increasing susceptibility to the common cold.
      c) By inflicting small cuts in volunteers who were then subjected to controlled stressful situations, researchers have shown a significant delay in healing among those under stress.
      d) People who were shown films of Mother Teresa consoling the poor and the sick experienced increased levels of Salivary Immunoglobulin A, one of the body's first lines of defense against invading pathogens. Children have been shown to be able to increase levels of this substance through relaxation and self-hypnosis, while humor has been shown to increase levels in adults.
      e) In research on women with metastatic breast cancer, psychiatrist David Spiegel found that stress hormones played a role in the progression of breast cancer. The average survival time of women with normal cortisol patterns was significantly longer than that of women whose cortisol levels remained high throughout the day (an indicator of stress).
   4. Candace Pert believes "The immune system, like the central nervous system has memory and the capacity to learn. Thus it can be said that intelligence is located not only in the brain but in cells that are distributed throughout the body, and that the traditional separation of mental processes, including emotions, from the body is no longer valid."

VII. **BLAMING THE VICTIM**
   A. In spite of our best efforts to manage stress and have a positive outlook on life, disease happens.
      1. The mentality that disease is the "fault" of the victim is not a productive approach to health.

2. A more constructive approach to health is to acknowledge that how we think and feel does have an impact on our health, yet some disease and death are inevitable.

VIII. CONCLUSION

A. Scientific studies provide a solid foundation of undeniable scientific evidence explaining the connection between the body and the mind.

B. Generalized and unabated stress places a person in a state of disequilibrium, which increases his or her susceptibility to a wide range of diseases and disorders.

C. There is no way to predict which maladies you will experience from too much stress in your life - there are too many factors involved.

1. Keeping the stress response activated increases your risk for many diseases and decreases the quality of your life.

2. A positive outlook can improve health.

LEARNING ACTIVITIES

ACTIVITY 1 - JOURNALING

Objective: The purpose of this activity is to encourage critical thinking and honest personal reflection on topics relating to the chapter content. Explore personal thoughts, feelings, values, and behaviors as you selectively incorporate stress management knowledge and behaviors into your plan for improved health through better stress management.

Instructions: You will find journaling questions in each chapter of your Activities Manual. These questions relate specifically to the chapter content. Moving your thoughts from your mind to the paper is a powerful strategy for relieving stress and for increasing awareness of your thoughts, feelings and behaviors. Your course instructor can provide further guidance on how to complete this activity.

Complete the following journaling questions. Select the questions that have the most relevance for you.

1. How do you think your thoughts can actually cause disease or cure disease? Explain your rationale.
2. Have you ever deliberately made yourself sick because you wanted to avoid a situation or event? Have you ever gotten sick at the end of a challenging semester or during a difficult time in your life? Explain how it makes sense that you were able to do this based on the information in this chapter.
3. Explain why the fight-or-flight response leads to the medium-term health effects of chronic stress.
4. Looking at the long-term effects of stress, why do you think we can say with confidence that stress impacts nearly every disease in our culture today?
5. Regarding psychoneuroimmunology, explain why two people could be in the same environment and only one of them catches a cold.
6. Explain why hardiness may be an important first step in preventing activation of the stress response.
7. How does the information in this chapter affect you personally? What insights did you have about yourself and the stress that you experience?

ACTIVITY 2 - HARMFUL HEALTH EFFECTS OF STRESS

Objectives: The purpose of this activity is to help you understand the effects of chronic stress in the short, medium and long-term.

Description of Activity: Begin this activity by writing two headings on a piece of paper: "short-term and medium-term effects of chronic stress" on the left side of the paper and "long-term effects of stress" on the right side. Using the information in the chapter and this outline, write examples of health problems associated with chronic stress and place them under the appropriate heading. List as many maladies as you can think of.

Start with short-term and medium-term effects of chronic stress. Think about the way that each malady is a result of chronic activation of the stress response. For example, a headache is usually the result of chronically tense muscles that go from the neck up and all around the head. Muscle pain works the same way. Insomnia results from thinking patterns that tell the body it should be doing something rather than resting.

Next, list long-term effects of stress. Make a list of diseases and conditions that are associated with stress. Nearly every disease in our culture has a stress component. Cancer is a good example of how this works: Everyone has cancer cells growing in their bodies, but the reason the cancer doesn't get the upper hand and cause too much damage is because our strong immune system keeps them in check. However, when the stress response is activated, the immune system is suppressed. If the immune system remains suppressed for a long period of time, it allows the cancer cells to grow more freely. The same explanation could be made with any pathogen, such as a virus or bacteria.

Always think of stress-related diseases in terms of what happens when the big bear emerges from the forest as depicted in the scenario in chapter 3. All diseases associated with stress are based on the premise that you need to run from or fight a big bear, but in our day there is no big bear. But when we perceive psychological danger the stress response is automatically turned on. Chronic activation of the fight-or-flight response leads to a chronic imbalance in nearly every system of the body. This leads to all the stress-related health problems.

ACTIVITY 3 – STRESS AND THE MIND/BODY CONNECTION

Objectives: The purpose of this activity is to help you see the detrimental health effects of stress using real world examples.

Description of Activity:
Find a research article or news story that involves an illness, malady, or disease. Considering information in chapter 4, select a health concern that has a stress component. In other words, there must be mention of stress as playing a part in the onset or progression of the health concern.

Search for your article or health news story using reputable health websites, magazines, or other appropriate health publications. Make a copy of the article or news story and bring it to class. With a partner or in a small group, discuss the contents of your news stories. Emphasize a focus on the stress component that contributed to the disease or poor health condition.

ACTIVITY 4 – THE PLACEBO EFFECT

Objectives: The purpose of this activity is to help you sense the power of the mind in creating health or illness via the placebo or nocebo effect.

Description of Activity:
The placebo effect occurs when a person believes that an inert substance (such as a sugar pill) has the power to create a specific health outcome (such as killing bacteria in the body or relieving pain), and the belief itself appears to be sufficient to bring about the hoped-for result. The opposite of the placebo effect is the nocebo effect in which sickness occurs as a result of believing with emotional intensity in an unhealthy outcome. Write your response to the following:
- Have you ever heard of someone who experienced the placebo or nocebo effect? If not, do some research to find an example. Describe what happened.
- We must be careful to not immediately assign every health problem to someone's poor way of thinking. Discuss the negative aspects of this 'blaming the victim' approach to health.
- Explain what might be considered more constructive scenarios to explain why a person struggles with a particular health challenge (perhaps a combination of nocebo as well as the presence of a pathogen).

ACTIVITY 5 – CHRONIC STRESS AND YOU

Objectives: The purpose of this activity is to help you see how chronic activation of the stress response can lead to health problems you may be experiencing.

Description of Activity:
Look at the list of health problems found in chapter 4 of the text in the section titled, **Effects of Medium-Term Chronic Stress.** Select a health condition that you experience from this list. Discuss the following points:
- Based on the information in chapters 3 and 4, explain how the problem probably occurs because of continued activation of the fight-or-flight response.
- Think of a condition that you or someone you know struggles with that is found in the section in chapter 4 of your text titled, **Other Disease Conditions of Stress.** Based on your understanding of the harmful effects of chronic activation of the stress response, explain why we can say with some confidence that stress is a contributing component in that adverse health condition.

RELATED WEBSITES

Mayo Clinic

Signs and symptoms of stress: Prompt recognition is crucial

http://www.mayoclinic.com/invoke.cfm?id=SR00008_D

Stress and Immunity

Great article on the effects of stress on the immune system – psychoneuroimmunology.

http://www.econ.uiuc.edu/%7Ehanko/Bio/stress.html

Stress: Signs and Symptoms, Causes and Effects

Excellent overview of the variety of symptoms of stress

http://www.helpguide.org/mental/stress_signs.htm

CHAPTER 5
THE POWER OF PERCEPTIONS

CHAPTER OUTLINE
Use this outline to take notes as you read the chapter in the text and/or as your instructor lectures in class.

I.   **THE POWER OF PERCEPTIONS**
   A.   There are many reasons why people react to things differently.
      1.   Genetics, perception, personality, or attitude and other reasons all play a part.
      2.   The most important reason that people respond differently is how they perceive or interpret the events.
      3.   A change in how you perceive things is the first critical step toward improving your stress experience.

II. **PERCEPTION**
   A.   A person's cognitive (mental) interpretation of events is perhaps the most important aspect in preventing unnecessary and unhealthy stress.
   B.   Ask yourself this very important question: In the past month of your life, how often did you find yourself in life-threatening situations?
      1.   We are very rarely in any kind of vital danger or at risk for physical pain from an outside source.
      2.   If we analyze our situations accurately, we will acknowledge that we typically do not live lives with many life-threatening experiences.
   C.   Refer back to the stress-o-meter self-assessment that you completed in Chapter 2.
      1.   Was your score higher than a 2 or 3?
      2.   If you are in real danger so infrequently, if you have so few genuinely threatening experiences where you need extra energy to survive, why would you report any score higher than 2 or 3 on the stress-o-meter?
         a)   Remember, the only purpose of the stress response is to keep you alive.
      3.   We are nearly always stressed over situations that are not, by their nature, sufficient to put us in real danger.
   D.   It is the perception or the interpretation of an event that initiates the fight-or-flight response. It is not the event itself that causes us to experience stress.
      1.   The notion that human stress is a direct response to external stimulus is no longer credible.
      2.   Whether we feel stressed appears to depend on how we view what is happening. Interpretation of stressors, not stressors themselves, causes distress.
      3.   Stress is a coupled action of the body and mind involving appraisal of a threat, an instant modulation of response.
         a)   The triggering mechanism is the individual's *perception* of threat, not an event.
   E.   Whenever we sense that there is a potential for pain or danger of any kind, emotional, social, spiritual, or physical, our body reacts in its perfect way to help us survive.
      1.   The only way the body knows to do this is to turn on the fight-or-flight response.
   F.   An exam or any other stressful event is only stressful because of how we interpret it.
III. **THE WORLD - A STRESSFUL PLACE OR NOT?**
   A.   No event in life is inherently stressful.
      1.   There is no event in life that causes stress universally for everyone.
         a)   We have decided that some aspect of the situation will inflict pain or discomfort, which may be physical, emotional, or spiritual.
   B.   This understanding shifts the influence of what causes us stress from external factors to internal control.
      1.   We have the power to take control of how we interpret any event in life.
      2.   When we experience stressful feelings, we are the sole cause.
         a)   Knowing this one single thing gives us complete power to undo those

stressful feelings.
       b) If we are feeling stress, we can immediately take responsibility for this experience and take positive measures to turn off the stress.
   C. We are not trained to think this way.
      1. From a very early age, we accept the mistaken belief that others have the power to make us feel certain ways.

IV. COGNITIVE RESTRUCTURING
   A. The mental act of changing the meaning or our interpretation of the environmental stressors in life.
      1. Also known as **reframing**.
      2. The approach substitutes our perceptions of stressors from thoughts that are threatening to thoughts that are non-threatening.
   B. When you approach life with a more accurate interpretation of events around you, not only does this positive perception halt the initiation of the stress response and the resulting disease and ill-health, but you also learn that you can turn problems into opportunities to reawaken your enthusiasm for life.

V. CONTROL
   A. A deeply held belief that you can directly impact a situation.
      1. There is a relationship between the amount of control we think we have and the corresponding amount of stress that we feel.
      2. The more control we feel we have over our circumstances, the less stress we tend to feel.
   B. There are some things in life over which we have no control.
      1. The stock market, the weather, other people, etc.
      2. The healthy response to things over which we have no control is acceptance, allowance, and a go-with-the-flow attitude.
   C. There are also things over which we have total control.
      1. Related to ourselves - our thoughts, feelings, and behaviors and actions.
        a) Nobody but you can control your inner life.
   D. There are some things over which we have more control than we believe.
      1. Many people have the faulty notion or belief that a person does not have the ability to carry out a specific task; this is called **self-limiting beliefs**.
      2. We tend to act on these beliefs and not achieve what we would like to.
      3. Argue for your limitations, and sure enough, they're yours.
        a) Our beliefs become our reality, regardless of their original accuracy.
        b) We tend to act on those limiting beliefs.
      4. If the need or desire is great enough, we can control a lot more than we think.
   E. **Locus of Control**
      1. Refers to the way that people ascribe their chances of success or failure in a future venture to either internal or external causes.
      2. People with an **internal locus of control** see themselves as responsible for the outcomes of their own actions.
        a) If your thinking is more toward the internal LOC end of the continuum you might say, "The grade I receive in this class is entirely dependant on the work, study, and effort I exert toward each of the assignments and tests."
      3. People with an **external locus of control** believe that whatever happens to them is unrelated to their own behavior, making it beyond their control.
        a) If you tend to think from a more external LOC perspective, you might think or say, "I will get a good grade in this class because the teacher likes me or is in a good mood when she is giving out grades."
      4. If you think you can control the stress that you are experiencing, you are well on your way to doing so.

5.

VI. SELF-EFFICACY

A. The belief in one's ability to accomplish a goal or change a behavior.

B. When we truly believe we can do something, we often find we can.

C. It isn't always easy, but people can and do take control of their thinking and their perceptions every day.

VII. PUTTING IT ALL TOGETHER

A. Anytime we find ourselves becoming tense, we can ask ourselves these questions:

1. **Is this stressor real?** Am I really in danger here or am I just imagining or creating the danger or pain?

    a) If we look at the situation with a rational eye, we find that rarely is the danger or pain real.

2. **Can I handle this situation?**

    a) Our past experience tells us that we can handle most potentially stressful situations successfully.

    b) Why should this one be any different?

3. **Can I think about this differently?**

    a) As an event happens, we have a choice about how we view it or what it means to us.

    b) Depending on how we interpret the situation will lead to feelings of calmness or stress.

VIII. CONCLUSION

A. These key points explain how your perceptions impacts stress:

1. Perception, or interpretation of events, determines the stress outcome.

2. Events are perceived as stressful if the expected outcome is threatening or painful.

3. We are actually in real danger less than 1 percent of the time; therefore, we rarely need the stress response for protection.

4. By changing how we interpret events, we can prevent the stress response from activating.

5. Preventing unnecessary stress will promote health, prevent disease, and improve the quality of your life.

LEARNING ACTIVITIES

ACTIVITY 1 - JOURNALING

Objective: The purpose of this activity is to encourage critical thinking and honest personal reflection on topics relating to the chapter content. Explore personal thoughts, feelings, values, and behaviors as you selectively incorporate stress management knowledge and behaviors into your plan for improved health through better stress management.

Instructions: You will find journaling questions in each chapter of your Activities Manual. These questions relate specifically to the chapter content. Moving your thoughts from your mind to the paper is a powerful strategy for relieving stress and for increasing awareness of your thoughts, feelings and behaviors. Your course instructor can provide further guidance on how to complete this activity.

Complete the following journaling questions. Select the questions that have the most relevance for you.

1. After reading this chapter, explain the statement, "It is not the event itself that causes us to experience stress." If it's not the event or situation, what is it that always causes us to feel stress? For example, why is your most challenging exam not really stressful?
2. Why do you think we can now say with some confidence, "The world is not a stressful place."
3. Where can you look to correctly answer the question, "Can I handle this situation?"
4. How does the information in this chapter affect you personally? What insights did you have about yourself and the stress that you experience?

ACTIVITY 2 - ARE YOU REALLY IN DANGER?

Objectives: The purpose of this discussion is to help you realize how infrequently you really have actual threats in your life.

Description of Activity: You will be doing some addition so you may need a calculator.
Start this activity by thinking of the previous month of your life - every waking moment. Next, think back to any events that you experienced in which your life was honestly in danger - or someone you were with was in danger. Situations like having an argument with parents or having to turn in a late assignment or anything of this nature are NOT life threatening (though you may have felt stress.) You are only looking for situations that are the equivalent of a situation where a big bear is running toward you.

As an example, you might say that you almost got hit by a car. The actual time that this took was probably 2 or 3 seconds in total. Everything else that occurred surrounding the incident such as the thoughts you had as you continued walking safely on your way home don't count. Only consider the time of the incident itself.

Thinking back over the past month, put the actual amount of time that was spent in life-threatening situations in the calculator and add them up. Your total will very likely be much less than 5 or 10 minutes of total time.

Next, do the following math:

First, you will figure the total number of minutes you lived last month: 30 (days) X 24 (hours in a day) X 60 (minutes in an hour). This will give you a number of 43,200 minutes that you lived last month.

Next, divide the accumulated number of minutes that were truly life-threatening into the total number of minutes you lived. Your results will calculate to less than 1%. In reality, very little of our lives are spent in situations that require the use of the stress response. We are very rarely in life-threatening situations.

Now ask yourself these two very important questions:

- In chapter 2, you completed several self-assessments. One of them was the Stress-O-Meter in which you gave yourself a general stress score of some number between 1 and 10 (10 being extremely high stress). Was the score that you gave yourself higher than a 2 or a 3?
- If you are so infrequently in situations that are life threatening, and since the stress response has only one function, which is to help you survive life threatening situations, why would you ever feel stress?

Take a few minutes to write down your thoughts and feelings as you consider these two questions.

ACTIVITY 3 - THE WORLD IS NOT A STRESSFUL PLACE

Objective: The purpose of this discussion is to help you realize that the real stressor of a situation is not usually what you think it is.

Description of Activity: Think of a situation in your mind that makes you feel uneasy, uncomfortable or stressed if you were to have to do it. A good example might be if you were asked to sing a song, like the National Anthem, in front of your class.

Think of a time when you went to a college or professional sporting event, like a basketball game. Recall what happens at the beginning of the game - at some point prior to the start of the game a person comes before the crowd and sings the Star Spangled Banner.

Imagine for a moment that you have been asked to sing the National Anthem in front of this large crowd assembled for the sporting event. Pretend that you are in front of the very large crowd before the start of the game. Imagine yourself holding a microphone and you are getting ready to sing.

Now think carefully. How would you feel if you were getting ready to sing this song? Would you feel nervous, anxious, scared, panicked?

Ask yourself and accurately answer the following questions:

- If you were to sing in front of this large group of people, would you feel stress?
- If you were at you house vacuuming or in your shower or doing dishes and you knew nobody was around to hear, would you have any problems singing the National Anthem?
- If you are doing virtually the same thing in both places - singing the same song with the same words with the same intensity - why would singing in front of the class feel so uncomfortable and singing at home wouldn't? Aren't you doing the same thing both places?
- Why would you feel stressed in one place and not the other doing the same thing?

Now ask yourself these questions:

- Is there ever any threat of pain or death while you are standing in front of this group of people singing (the correct answer is no)?
- If you were never in any danger, what was it about your experience that made you feel stressed in front of the large audience?

We learn from this example that it is rarely the situation or the event that causes us to feel stress, but it is instead the way we interpret what is happening. The world is not a stressful place, there are only stressful interpretations of a world that is by and large unthreatening. There are exceptions, but as we discovered earlier, these happen far less than one percent of the time.

ACTIVITY 4 - DISCOVERING THE POINT OF PAIN

Objectives: The purpose of this activity is to help you discover what the real pain or discomfort is in a situation or event you find stressful.

Materials needed:
Handout 5:1 - Discovering the Point of Pain

Description of Activity: Complete Handout 5:1 - Discovering the Point of Pain according to the instructions.

Handout 5:1 - Discovering the Point of Pain

Name _____

Nearly every stress that you feel involves the thought of pain that you must prepare for and try to avoid. This assignment is an investigation to find out where that pain really is.

Think of a situation or event that you find very stressful - one that you personally experienced or are experiencing now. Write that experience or event below.

Next, follow through the steps of that event or situation and analyze it from beginning to its natural end. Assess where any real pain happens during each step. Do not include psychological pain that you make up about it, but just describe the real physical pain that happened to you or is currently happening.

Finally, analyze each step of the event and follow it through to the imagined point where you feel there might be pain. For example, if you didn't do so well on a test, what *real* pain have you imagined might happen? Follow this through to its logical end in your mind. Then transfer it to the space below.

1. List the stressful event or situation

2. What real pain has occurred or is occurring?

3. Write the steps that lead to the pain, and the *final real pain* that you are trying to avoid (For example, if you do poorly on a test, this may lead to not getting a good grade, which may lead to not getting a scholarship, which may lead to ... etc.)

4. Assess the likelihood that the *real* pain that you imagine might happen really will. For example, if the real pain of doing poorly on a test is losing your scholarship, assess the real likelihood of that happening.

Once you do this, you immediately diffuse the need to activate the stress response because you realize you are safe rather than threatened by some unlikely future pain for which you need to prepare.

RELATED WEBSITES

Perception: A Key Variable in Family Stress Management
Communication, problem-solving, decision-making, and stress management are all greatly affected by the perception of the individuals and families involved. That is, they make some sense or meaning of it; they interpret; they define situations and events; they make inferences and draw conclusions.
http://www.extension.umn.edu/distribution/familydevelopment/DE2776.html

Cognitive Restructuring - From Unhappiness to a Positive Outlook...
Our moods are driven by what we tell ourselves, and this is usually based on our interpretations of our environment. Cognitive Restructuring helps us evaluate how rational and valid these interpretations are.
http://www.mindtools.com/stress/rt/CognitiveRestructuring.htm

Reframing
Reframing is a technique used to change the way you look at things in order to feel better about them.
http://www.mentalhealth.com/mag1/p51-str.html#Head_1g

CHAPTER 6
THINKING AND CHOOSING

CHAPTER OUTLINE
Use this outline to take notes as you read the chapter in the text and/or as your instructor lectures in class.

I. THINKING AND CHOOSING
    A. The stress you are feeling begins with a thought.
        1. Your thoughts shape the events and circumstances of your life.
        2. Cognitive (thinking) techniques help change stress-producing thought patterns into thought patterns that can actually prevent stress.
II. COGNITIVE DISTORTIONS
    A. **Cognitive distortion** occurs when thoughts are magnified out of proportion to their seriousness, resulting in excess stress.
    B. Examples of cognitive distortions:
        1. All-or-nothing thinking.
            a) Everything is seen as an extreme (good or bad), so there is no middle ground.
        2. Personalizing
            a) The tendency to assume responsibility for things that are out of your control.
        3. Discounting the positive
            a) Many people feel they are undeserving of praise so they choose to not accept a compliment.
        4. Assuming the worst
            a) Also called pessimism or awfulizing.
            b) Looking forward and deciding that the future will not bring good outcomes.
    C. Distortions in thinking often lead to feelings that are associated with stress.
        1. **Cognitive therapy** is intended to focus on cognitive distortions and the relearning of thought processes as a way to alter negative emotions such as depression, to raise self-esteem, and to gain hope for the future.
III. THINKING ERRORS
    A. Psychologist Albert Ellis identified twelve irrational ideas he calls "thinking errors" that are common to our culture.
        1. These beliefs and conditioned responses often take the form of absolute statements. (See Chart - 12 Irrational Ideas that Create and Add to Stress).
        2. Changing irrational ideas to a more rational disputing idea can immediately prevent the associated unpleasant emotions that tend to follow the irrational idea.
IV. COGNITIVE TECHNIQUES THAT HELP OVERCOME DISTORTED THINKING
    A. Positive Self Talk
        1. **Self-talk**, also known as our **stream of consciousness**, describes the messages you send to yourself, your internal dialogue.
            a) Becoming aware of this stream of consciousness and listening to what you are thinking is the first step in mastering your self-talk.
            b) Many of us don't even realize how often our self-talk is negative.
            c) Much of the internal dialogue in the mind occurs as a result of habit.
                (1) With frequent repetition of any negative judgment about ourselves, we begin to believe it.
                (2) You can change how you feel about yourself by talking to yourself like you would to a friend you care about.
        2. Think about a recent experience where you felt angry or frustrated.
            a) Describe your self-talk during the event.
            b) Now try rethinking the whole situation using positive self-talk.

      c) Positive self-talk can improve self-esteem and eliminate the chronic, nagging stress that destroys people from the inside out.

B. **Thought Stopping**
1. Stopping negative thoughts when they enter your stream of consciousness.
   a) When an unconstructive thought creeps into your mind, recognize your choice to think, and say "STOP."
   b) Replace the stress-producing, negative statement with a positive statement.
2. The outcome of positive self-talk and thought stopping is **learned optimism**.

C. **Power Language**
1. A way of speaking that helps you boost your feeling of control simply by changing the words you use.
   a) Compare these two statements:
      (1) "I can't handle this deadline."
      (2) "I won't handle this deadline."
   b) "I won't" is a choice you make - an act of will - resulting in a sense of control rather than helplessness.
2. Anthony Robbins said, "Simply by changing your habitual vocabulary - the words you consistently use to describe the emotions of your life - you can instantaneously change how you think, how you feel, and how you live."
   a) Refer to Table 6.1 to see suggestions for making slight adjustments to our internal conversations.

D. **Going with the Flow**
1. Acceptance of situations we can not control.
2. We tend to overlook acceptance because it can be difficult.
3. If you can't fight it or flee it ... flow with it.

V. **UNDERLYING THEORIES AND TECHNIQUES**
A. **Conditioned response theory** proposes that when things happen in our environment, we are conditioned to respond in certain ways.
1. Russian physiologist Ivan Pavlov conducted a series of experiments dealing with salivation responses in dogs.
   a) Pavlov would introduce a stimulus of food to a dog, and immediately the dog would salivate.
      (1) This is a natural response.
   b) Pavlov then introduced a sound (he used various sounds such as whistles and tuning forks) simultaneously with the introduction of the food.
      (1) The dog still responded with salivation with the introduction of that paired stimulus - the food and the sound.
   c) Finally, he introduced the sound but now without the presence of the food.
      (1) The dog was conditioned to salivate to the sound because it associated the sound with the food.
2. We are conditioned to a very large degree.
   a) Many of our learned behaviors serve us well.
   b) Other patterns of behavior (conditioned responses) that we perform automatically do not serve us quite so well.
      (1) For example, when someone is yelling obscenities at us, we get angry, offended, and defensive.
      (2) These are conditioned or learned responses. They are not inherited tendencies.
   c) If we learned to respond in a particular way to something that happens, we can also unlearn it.

B. **Choice**
1. We have the capacity to place something between stimulus and response that immediately puts us in control of how that situation will affect us.

         a) That important element is choice.

     2. In any situation, we have the power to choose our response to what is happening.

         a) We do not automatically have to react with anger toward the person who is yelling at us.

         b) We can choose to remain calm, to turn and walk away, or to return this person's anger with our own.

     3. Victor Frankl tells of one of the most profound examples of how we can be responsible (response-able) for our thoughts and feelings in his book *Man's Search for Meaning.*

         a) He came to realize that regardless of what his Nazi captors did to him, he had total and complete choice of how he would respond.

             (1) Whenever we are upset, angry, bored, nervous, anxious, embarrassed, shy, or experience any other emotion, it is because of our thoughts, and not the event .

VI. LEVELS OF RESPONDING

    A. Things happen in our days over which we have absolutely no control.

     1. When we notice these uncontrollable events, there is a tendency to react before we think about how we are reacting. We are on autopilot.

     2. While individuals respond to events in a variety of ways, we can categorize how people respond to uncontrollable events in two broad categories, *effective responding* and *ineffective responding.* (Refer to Table 6.2 Levels of Responding).

         a) We call them effective or ineffective based on if they result in feelings associated with relaxation such as joy, peace of mind, balance, growth and happiness or if they result in emotions such as anger, fear, frustration, imbalance, boredom, and chaos.

    B. Ineffective Responding - Below the Line

     1. Attachment/Rightness

         a) When we become emotionally attached to ideas and situations, we think that we know what is best and cling emotionally to that view.

         b) When we attach ourselves to opinions, ideas, and how we think things "ought to be," we find ourselves in arguments, we mistrust other people who do not think as we do, and we are disappointed when our expectations aren't met.

     2. Judgment/Criticism/Blaming

         a) The mental act of putting a label on something and then trying to make that label the reality.

             (1) People who react in this way tend to judge and criticize things, people, circumstances, and situations.

             (2) It is impossible to accurately judge a situation or a person based on limited experiences.

             (3) When we judge, we have essentially closed off other possible ways of seeing that person or situation.

             (4) When we judge, we are trying to elevate our worth to a higher level than the person we are judging.

         b) The resulting feelings we experience when we respond judgmentally or critically to situations are guilt, shame, low self-worth, and false pride.

     3. Resistance

         a) The mental process of wishing things were different than they are.

         b) The problem with this thought is that often things cannot be different than they are.

         c) There are several ways to notice if we are resisting what is happening.

             (1) Anger

             (2) Feeling tired or bored

             (3) If we notice that time is moving very slowly during an event, we

are probably resisting it.

- C. Effective Responding - Above the Line
    1. Observation
        a) The simple act of noticing something without adding anything.
        b) Our senses bring us data from the outside world and we simply become aware.
        c) We are just taking in the information that presents itself.
            (1) We might respond by saying something like "Hmm..." or "I am noticing or observing ... (whatever my senses bring into my awareness)."
    2. Discovery
        a) Focuses on observation and adds an additional component of learning, of seeking to understand, of discovery.
        b) We observe what is happening and we seek to find out what we can learn from it.
        c) We live in the questioning mode.
    3. Allowance and Acceptance.
        a) Emotionally embracing what is happening as the way things are and we are okay with them.
        b) Acceptance is realizing that what is happening is how it is and it isn't any other way ... and that is okay.
    4. Gratitude
        a) Witnessing an event and showing appreciation or thankfulness for the opportunity of experiencing this moment.
        b) We see each moment as a gift that will help us grow, develop and enjoy life even more.
    5. When we respond above the line, we remain in greater control of our inner environment, and as a result, we prevent stress from happening.
        a) We are in charge of our inner life regardless of what is happening outside of us.
- D. The way we respond to the events in life results in either an empowering proactive attitude or a disempowering, reactive attitude.
    1. We are typically not conditioned to respond at the more effective levels.
    2. If we respond ineffectively, we create a chaotic inner environment that will activate the stress response.

VII. RATIONAL EMOTIVE BEHAVIOR THERAPY
- A. Stress-related behaviors are initiated by self-defeating perceptions that can be changed.
- B. REBT emphasizes replacing defeating, victimizing thoughts and feelings with more accurate and powerful thoughts.
- C. REBT is based on these principles:
    1. You are responsible for your own emotions and actions.
    2. Your harmful emotions and dysfunctional behaviors are the product of your own irrational thinking.
    3. You can learn more realistic views and, with practice, make them a part of you.
    4. You will experience a deeper acceptance of yourself and greater satisfactions in life by developing a reality-based perspective.
- D. According to REBT, there are two different types of difficulties:
    1. **Practical problems**
        a) Relate to such things as events that result in feelings of being treated unfairly by others or being in undesirable situations.
        b) These are usually experiences over which you have little, if any, control.
        c) This emotional disturbance unnecessarily creates a second order of problems - emotional suffering.
    2. **Emotional problems**

a) Disturbances over which you have total control.
   E. REBT Guidelines: You begin taking control, and minimizing emotional suffering, by
      following these guidelines:
      1. Take responsibility for your emotional upsets and distress.
         a) Only you can upset yourself about events - the events themselves, no
            matter how undesirable, can never upset you. They do not have this power.
      2. Identify your "musts."
         a) Determine what you are demanding of yourself, of other people in your
            life, or of your life's circumstances.
         b) Once you have figured what the "must" is behind your emotion, you are
            then able to move forward and effectively reduce your distress.
      3. Determine the reality of your "musts."
         a) Ask yourself: "What is the evidence for my *must*?" "How is it true?" "Where
            is it etched in stone?"
         b) And then by seeing: "There is no evidence." "My *must* is entirely false." "It
            is not carved indelibly anywhere." Make your view *must-free* and your
            emotions will heal.
      4. Upgrade your "musts" to preferences.
         a) Change your thoughts about what "must" happen to "I prefer that this
            happen."
   F. ABCDE Technique: Examining irrational beliefs that make us anxious, changing those
      beliefs, and envisioning more positive consequences of our actions based on the ABCDE
      technique that includes the following steps:
      1. A. Activating event (identify the stressor)
      2. B. Belief system (identify rational and irrational beliefs)
      3. C. Consequences (mental, physical, behavioral)
      4. D. Dispute irrational beliefs
      5. E. Effect (change consequences).
   G. When an activating event (A) occurs, it can cause a reaction or consequence (C) in a
      person. However, after careful examination, we may find that A did not, in fact, cause C.
      The thing that really caused C to happen was the person's belief system (B).
   H. Successfully dispute (D) the irrational thought.
      1. You can change your way of thinking to a more accurate series of thoughts.
   I. Once we dispute (D) the irrational belief, we are now free to enjoy the positive
      psychological effects (E) of the more rational belief.

VIII.   CONCLUSION
   A. How we think matters! What you think creates how you feel.
   B. Managing our self-talk, stopping negative thoughts, and going with the flow are powerful
      mental tools to help us prevent activation of the stress response.
   C. Awareness of our levels of responding, rational emotive behavior therapy, and other
      cognitive techniques introduced in this chapter can help you take control of your thoughts
      and help you experience inner peace.

LEARNING ACTIVITIES

ACTIVITY 1 – JOURNALING

Objective: The purpose of this activity is to encourage critical thinking and honest personal reflection on topics relating to the chapter content. Explore personal thoughts, feelings, values, and behaviors as you selectively incorporate stress management knowledge and behaviors into your plan for improved health through better stress management.

Instructions: You will find journaling questions in each chapter of your Activities Manual. These questions relate specifically to the chapter content. Moving your thoughts from your mind to the paper is a powerful strategy for relieving stress and for increasing awareness of your thoughts, feelings and behaviors. Your course instructor can provide further guidance on how to complete this activity.

Complete the following journaling questions. Select the questions that have the most relevance for you.

1. What are some common words that you use that could be changed to more empowering ones, such as replacing "can't" for "won't" or "choose not to?"
2. In the Thinking Errors section of the chapter, find two thinking error patterns or irrational thoughts that you commonly notice about yourself. How could you change that way of thinking to be more effective and rational?
3. Why is it, in reality, impossible to be offended by something someone else says or does?
4. What do you think is the essence of Viktor Frankl's comment on the last of the human freedoms?
5. Carefully read through the levels of responding section. As you do, think of a situation in which you experienced anger, frustration, anxiety, boredom or some other unpleasant feeling. Similar to the author anecdote where you read about the author's experience riding a bike and getting garbage thrown at him, go through each of the levels of responding and describe what you might say to yourself that would result in peacefulness and no stress rather than responding ineffectively and feeling an unpleasant emotion.
6. How does the information in this chapter affect you personally? What insights did you have about yourself and the stress that you experience?

ACTIVITY 2 – CHOOSING TO RESPOND MORE EFFECTIVELY

Objectives: The purpose of this activity is to give you a clearer view of how you can choose to respond to situations in more effective, less stressful ways.

Materials needed:
Handout 6:1 - Level of Responding Chart, Handout 6:2 - Levels of Responding Worksheet, pen or pencil

Duration of Activity: 25-30 minutes

Description of Activity: Recall a situation in which you recently found yourself experiencing an unpleasant emotion: anger, frustration, boredom, or guilt for example. Notice which of the ways listed in the Levels of Responding Chart describe how you were responding to what was happening, for example, getting angry because things weren't happening the way you thought they should.

Take a moment and relive the situation or event and describe how you could have responded differently based on the effective ways of responding on the chart. Describe what might have happened had you responded in the above-the-line ways and how you would have felt emotionally as a result of responding more effectively.

Complete Handout 6:2 - Levels of Responding Worksheet.

Handout 6:1 Levels of Responding Chart

Usefulness	Degree of Inner Peace	Ways We Respond to Events	Sounds Like (what we say to ourselves)	How We feel – What We Get – Our Resulting Emotional State
Effective: Leads to feelings associated with relaxation	More Peace	Gratitude	I appreciate …	Joy, serenity, contentment
		Allowance/Acceptance	It's okay … I embrace … I can live with this … I can go with the flow	Peace, release, relaxation, freedom
		Discovery	I wonder … What would happen if…? What can I learn from this?	Inquisitiveness, curiosity, growth
		Observation	I am noticing …	Calm
Ineffective: Leads to feelings associated with stress	Less Peace	Resistance/Complaining	I wish things were different (complaining)	Boredom, fatigue, anger
		Judgment/Criticism/Blaming	This is really a /He is really a (insert a negative noun) …	Guilt, shame, low self-worth, false pride
		Attachment/Rightness	This *must* be a certain way… Use words like must, have to, need to, should have	Mistrust, anxiety, anger, disappointment

Handout 6:2 Worksheet on Levels of Responding

Think of a situation that you encounter occasionally that tends to cause you to feel stressed.
Write it down here:

_____

Go through each way that you could respond to that situation and how you could see the situation differently by reconstructing your thoughts according to the table below:

Ways We Respond to Events	Sounds Like (what we say to ourselves)	What you might say to yourself
Gratitude	I appreciate …I'm thankful for …	
Allowance/Acceptance	It's okay … I embrace … I can live with this … I can go with the flow	
Discovery	I wonder … What would happen if…? What can I learn from this?	
Observation	I am noticing …	
Resistance/Complaining	I wish things were different (complaining)	
Judgment/Criticism/ Blaming	This is really a /He is really a (insert a negative noun) …	
Attachment/Rightness	This *must* be a certain way… Use words like must, have to, need to, should have	

ACTIVITY 3 - A DAY ABOVE THE LINE

Objectives: The purpose of this activity is to allow you to practice for an entire day responding to situations in ways that are more peaceful and less stressful.

Materials needed:
Handout 6:3 - A Day Above the Line

Description of Activity: Complete Handout 6:3 - A Day Above the Line. Follow the instructions as they are outlined on the handout.

HANDOUT 6:3 - A DAY ABOVE THE LINE

To complete this exercise, you are going to spend an entire day focusing on the principle of present moment acceptance and responding to every situation in ways that are above the line (See the Levels of Responding Chart). Amidst all of your other activities of the day, you will keep in mind a constant awareness of the more effective ways of responding to people, situations, and experiences (noticing, discovering, accepting/allowing, and appreciating). You will work to avoid responding to situations ineffectively (judging, criticizing, being right, and resisting). You might use some type of cue to remind you to focus on your thinking. This may be a rubber band on your wrist, a particular shirt, or some other unique item suitable for the day to be used to bring to your mind your direction of focus. Try to do this on a busy day when there are a lot of things going on.

At the end of the day that you choose to do this, describe your experience by writing about it using your computer. Write about opportunities you had to choose between effective and ineffective responding. Write what happened. Describe what you noticed about your sense of inner peace, harmony and happiness. Describe challenges and insights.

ACTIVITY 4 - CHANGING ERRONEOUS THINKING

Objectives: The purpose of this activity is to help you see ways to change common erroneous ways of thinking to more effective ways.

Materials needed:
Handout 6:4 - Changing Erroneous Thinking
Pen or pencil

Duration of Activity: 10 minutes

Description of Activity: Refer to information in chapter 6 to help you with this exercise. Follow the directions provided on Handout 6:4 - Changing Erroneous Thinking.

Handout 6:4 Changing Erroneous Thinking

Look at these erroneous types of thinking. Give a real world example and then give an appropriate, more rational and effective thought to take its place.

1. **Jumping to conclusions** - without evidence to back it up.
    a. example:

    b. better thought:

2. **Dualistic thinking** - interpreting a mild rebuff as a total rejection.
    a. example:

    b. better thought:

3. **Over-generalizing** - concluding from one mistake that we'll never do anything right.
    a. example:

    b. better thought:

4. **Errors of omission** - emphasizing a detail while ignoring its larger context.
    a. example:

    b. better thought:

5. **Personalizing** - taking something personally that isn't intended that way.
    a. example:

    b. better thought:

6. **Awfulizing** - nothing is just bad – it's horrible!
    a. example:

    b. better thought:

7. **Rationalizing -** opposite of awfulizing - deny feelings and under react.
    a. example:

    b. better thought:

8. **Pessimism** - looking at the worst in situations.
    a. example:

    b. better thought:

9. **Polarized thinking** - everything is viewed as good/bad, right/wrong, no middle ground.
    a. example:

    b. better thought:

10. **Should-ing** - reprimanding self for things you think you should have done.
    a. example:

    b. better thought:

ACTIVITY 5 - SELF-TALK

Objectives: The purpose of this activity is to help you recognize and change your own self-talk to be more positive and stress-relieving.

Materials: Handout 6:5 – Self-Talk Exercise

Instructions: Refer to the information in Chapter 6 on self-talk. Complete Handout 6:5 – Self-Talk Exercise to help you listen to, and make positive changes, to your accustomed way of thinking.

Handout 6:5 Self-Talk Exercise

Think of the mind as a tape player. We push the play button and the same old thoughts that we had yesterday are played again today. Frequently, we play mental tapes that reflect thoughts of negativity, weakness, and low self-esteem. These tapes often include the constant repetition of many negative words such as the following: "no, can't, won't, maybe, never, I can't, if only I ..., I don't know, I ought to, I should, I need to, etc.

Bring to mind a situation or event in which your thoughts included some of these words about yourself. In detail, write about this situation here:

Now, think of how you could select a different tape to listen to which would feed more positive messages into your subconscious mind. Consider using such positive words as these: I no longer, I am, I can, I will, I do.

How could you change your self-talk in this situation above so that you would act powerfully instead of weakly? Proactively instead of reactively? Peacefully instead of fearfully? Use the following space to write this new empowering tape:

ACTIVITY 6 – AS A MAN THINKETH

Objectives: The purpose of this activity is to expose you to a classic writer who clearly explains the principles outlined in this chapter.

Materials needed:
Handout 6:6 – As a Man Thinketh; the book titled "As a Man Thinketh.

Description of Activity: Follow the instructions provided on Handout 6:6 – As a Man Thinketh

Handout 6:6 As a Man Thinketh

This assignment involves reading the classic little book on thinking by James Allen titled, "As a Man Thinketh."

While you are reading it, and after you are finished, you will respond to the following items:

- What are the main ideas James Allen wanted us to consider in this book?
- What passages of the book had the most impact on you with respect to thoughts? Include them in your paper.
- What did James Allen feel were the means for reducing stress and correcting our thoughts? Be thorough in your thoughts about this one.
- What points of the book did you find particularly useful for decreasing your own stress levels and achieving mental and emotional wellness?
- Include in your work at least one quote from the book that had an impact on you as you read it. After the quote, explain why you felt the way you did about it.

Answer these questions in a typed format. Be sure to include your name at the top of your work.

The following are simple ways for you to get your hands on this marvelous volume.

You can buy it cheaply in a bookstore or check it out from the library.

It is also freely available online:

From this site, you can download an e-book version and have it immediately on your computer screen:
http://asamanthinketh.net/

From this site, and many others like it, you may read it directly from the website:
http://website.lineone.net/~jamesallen1/think.htm

You can also have the book sent directly to you via regular mail from this website:
http://www.changethatsrightnow.com/as_a_man_request.asp

Enjoy!

RELATED WEBSITES

Challenging irrational ideas (Rational-Emotive therapy)
Rational-Emotional therapy is built on the belief that how we emotionally respond at any moment depends on our interpretations--our views, our beliefs, our thoughts--of the situation. In other words, the things we think and say to ourselves, not what actually happens to us, cause our positive or negative emotions.
http://mentalhelp.net/psyhelp/chap14/chap14g.htm

Self-Talk & Self-Health
An article by Julia E. Weikle on how individuals can tap into the power of their own self-talk by recognizing it for what it is, reducing harmful negativity, and increasing the number of positive internal messages.
http://reading.indiana.edu/ieo/digests/d84.html

Thinkarete Notes on Learned Optimism
We all know that optimists see the glass as half-full while pessimists see it as half-empty. But, that doesn't come close to doing justice to the importance of optimism and how it affects our lives.
http://www.thinkarete.com/wisdom/works/notes/1429/

CHAPTER 7
MINDFULNESS

CHAPTER OUTLINE

Use this outline to take notes as you read the chapter in the text and/or as your instructor lectures in class.

I. THE NATURE OF REALITY
    A. This focus on mindfulness begins with a look at reality.
        1. **Reality** is what is ... what is happening.
        2. **Unreality** is what is not ... what is not happening.
        3. We can tell what is happening through our senses.
        4. We can also tell what is happening by the sensations we have internally.
        5. Reality, in essence, is what we experience.
        6. What is not reality are the things that we make up, our judgments, our opinions or ideas *about* our experience

II. THE HERE AND NOW.
    A. Here and now is all there is.
        1. Next focus looks at here and now.
            a) You are always right here.
                (1) It is never otherwise.
            b) You are always in the moment of right now.
                (1) It is never otherwise.
        2. Every moment of our life is successive moments of here and now.
    B. Experiencing here and now moments is the basis of mindfulness.

III. UNDERSTANDING MINDFULNESS
    A. **Mindfulness** is commonly defined as the state of being attentive to and aware of what is taking place in the present.
        1. It is a conscious discipline that can be explained as the intentional cultivation of non-judgmental moment-to-moment awareness.
            a) It is not so much a technique as a way of life.
            b) Mindfulness approaches are not considered relaxation techniques, but rather a form of mental training to reduce vulnerability to reactive modes of thinking that heighten stress and emotional distress.
            c) Mindfulness is based on the ancient contemplative tradition called **vipassana**, which means "seeing clearly."
            d) Mindfulness is the process of learning how to be with all experiences while being less judgmental and reactive.
            e) **Mindlessness** occurs when our thoughts are not in the present moment and when we tune out what is happening.
                (1) Our mental focus is on times and places other than here and now.
                (2) We ignore the present moment because our attention is focused elsewhere.

IV. QUALITIES OF MINDFULNESS
    A. Beginner's Mind - Thinking like a child
        1. This quality relates to the openness with which experiences are observed.
        2. Involves the quality of seeing things "as if for the first time," a quality that is often referred to as "beginner's mind."
            a) This means to look at the present moment, see what's in it, and experience it fully.
    B. Non-judging
        1. This quality represents straightforward observation.
            a) It means that one should not infer from what one is observing, and should not evaluate the observation in any way.
            b) We do this by simply staying in an observational state of mind without

judgment and expectations called **detached observation.**
   - c) Think of it like the mind being a wide movie screen with your thoughts projected on the screen.
      - (1) You observe them without judgment or analysis.
      - (2) The result is often increased awareness.

C. Acceptance of what is happening
   1. It is attending to and allowing what is happening now.
      - a) To bring our focus more into the present, simply turn off the mind chatter that is racing through our minds of what is not happening; about the future and the past, about thinking we always need to be somewhere else, about our opinions, judgments, and things we make up about an event.
   2. We can also simply attend to *what is* with all of our senses.
      - a) We observe, we notice, we watch, we become sensory-aware of what is happening in our environment.
      - b) When we notice ourselves getting wrapped up in our thoughts, we simply step back and let the moments unfold, observing and not trying to change anything.

D. Non-attachment
   1. The observer is detached from the object.
   2. This process of letting go is an important aspect of mindfulness that involves resisting the need to cling emotionally to anything.
      - a) We give up the need for things to be a certain way.
      - b) We let things be as they are.

E. Non-striving
   1. Implies giving up our need to try to change anything.
   2. We are no longer doing, we are just being.
   3. We let go of our need to *do* anything.
   4. We are just content with *being.*

V. **MINDFULNESS AS A WAY OF BEING**
   A. Mindfulness can be practiced in all aspects of daily life by bringing awareness to all activities and to all experiences.
      1. Mindfulness in daily life simply means to be present in all of one's activities and interactions.
      2. When we live mindfully, focusing our attention on what is happening here and now, and allowing ourselves to be totally absorbed in the activity at hand, we become more effective and productive, whatever the task, be it skiing down a tricky slope or doing our best on a tough test.
         - a) As we do this, in as many moments as possible, we begin to understand the fact that there is no other moment in time or point in space but that which is happening here and now.

VI. **WHY BE MINDFUL?**
   A. Focusing on the moment helps to clear the mind of clutter.
      1. As our thoughts of future and past accumulate, our minds get cluttered, and the result is **sensory overload.**
         - a) Sensory overload is like a blackboard filled to capacity with notes, scribbles, and information that is difficult to organize and understand.
         - b) A cluttered mind becomes a stressed mind.
         - c) Practicing mindfulness is like cleaning the mind's blackboard with an eraser. Mindfulness unclutters the mind and brings about mental tranquility.
   B. The greatest lapses in concentration come when we allow our minds to project what is about to happen or to dwell on what has already happened.
   C. There is no stress in the present moment.
      1. Stress only occurs for us when we allow our minds to think of other things besides

what is happening in our current experience.
2. We focus our thoughts on potential future events, about the past, and about things that might be happening elsewhere.
   a) When we associate any kind of pain or discomfort with those thoughts of other times and places, we initiate the stress response as a natural reaction to the perception of a false emergency.
3. Mindfulness turns off the stress response, and as a result, facilitates relaxation, reduces stress hormones, and boosts the immune system.

VII. **BENEFITS OF MINDFULNESS**
A. When we turn our mental focus exclusively to what is happening in the present moment, the stress response turns off.
1. You can test this principle by focusing all of the senses directly on something that is in your immediate environment.
2. When we focus our attention on what is happening, when we keep our awareness on here and now, what we get is an experience without stress.

VIII. **EXPERIENCING MINDFULNESS: TESTING THE PRINCIPLE**
A. When we focus our attention on what is happening, when we keep our awareness on the here and now, what we get is an experience without stress.
B. Practice by focusing directly on your hand to the exclusion of everything else.
1. When you do this as described in the chapter, what you get is stress -free moments.

IX. **INNER MINDFULNESS MEDITATION**
A. Inner mindfulness meditation, also called thought-watching, focuses the mind internally rather than externally through the five senses.
1. One's awareness is not limited to any one focal point, but is allowed to view one's thoughts as one would view a movie that is happening inside one's own mind, from a detached observational perspective.

X. **A SIMPLE MINDFUL EXERCISE**
A. This activity involves practicing being mindful for about 45 minutes to an hour. (Follow the Full Mindfulness Activity later in this chapter of this instructor's manual to complete this activity.)

XI. **MINDFULNESS SELF-EFFICACY**
A. **Mindfulness self-efficacy** relates to the question: How confident are you that your ability to maintain moment-to-moment non-judgmental awareness will keep you peaceful?
1. Imagine yourself in these or other situations where you might experience stress.
2. Think deliberately about how you can apply mindfulness to that situation by simple observing and being aware, rather than reacting in a stress-producing way.
3. Imagine how different your experience with stress will be.
4. As you practice mindfulness and apply it in your daily life, your self-efficacy will increase.

XII. **WAYS TO PRACTICE BEING MORE MINDFUL**
A. Choose an activity that you do in a less than mindful way and focus on involving yourself completely in the experience.
B. Pay attention to things that are happening around you.
C. Consciously speak to yourself, saying something like, "In this moment, I allow myself to be here now. I cannot be anywhere else right now nor can I be in my past or future, so I might as well relax and enjoy what is happening, here and now."
D. Take mindfulness breaks in which you do nothing but be totally engaged in a particular place and time.
E. Try a new sport or hobby. Totally engage yourself in learning a new skill.
F. Slightly change your normal routines.
G. When you are involved in, or notice others engaging in situations with heightened emotion, step back and simply become an observer rather than becoming emotionally involved in the incident.

XIII. **PLANNING FOR THE FUTURE**
   A. It is important to clarify that mindfulness does *not* mean living with reckless abandon *for the moment*.
      1. It means living fully *in the moment*.
   B. What are we to do about planning, setting goals, and creating our own futures?
      1. Planning for the future and creating goals is the process of bringing future moments into the present so appropriate control can be made toward achieving them.
         a) When we plan something we use our imagination constructively to create a future reality.
      2. Worrying about the future and putting our focus on the potentially painful outcomes of a future event is not productive.
         a) Worry happens when we think of a future event and then imagine possible outcomes of the events that include the potential for some kind of pain or discomfort that we would prefer avoiding.

XIV. **PUTTING IT ALL TOGETHER**
   A. Think of mindfulness in two stages.
      1. The first stage focuses on the self-regulation of attention so that it is maintained on immediate experience.
      2. The second stage involves adopting a particular orientation toward one's experiences in the present moment, an orientation that is characterized by curiosity, openness, and acceptance.

XV. **CONCLUSION**
   A. The ability to enjoy the present moment, mindfulness, is one of the essentials for stress management.
      1. To be at peace with oneself, learn to replace thoughts that produce unhealthy emotions like guilt, worry, fear, and anger, with a mental focus on the present.
      2. There are thousands of moments within the day to focus directly on the here and now moment.

<u>LEARNING ACTIVITIES</u>

ACTIVITY 1 - JOURNALING

Objective: The purpose of this activity is to encourage critical thinking and honest personal reflection on topics relating to the chapter content. Explore personal thoughts, feelings, values, and behaviors as you selectively incorporate stress management knowledge and behaviors into your plan for improved health through better stress management.

Instructions: You will find journaling questions in each chapter of your Activities Manual. These questions relate specifically to the chapter content. Moving your thoughts from your mind to the paper is a powerful strategy for relieving stress and for increasing awareness of your thoughts, feelings and behaviors. Your course instructor can provide further guidance on how to complete this activity.

Complete the following journaling questions. Select the questions that have the most relevance for you.

1. What does it mean to be mindful? How can you incorporate this in your life?
2. There is the example in the chapter of a person taking a test and a person shooting a foul shot. Give another similar example that clearly demonstrates why it is not the event, but how you are thinking about the event, that causes stress.
3. Summarize your understanding of what Thich Nhat Hanh said about washing dishes and the following author anecdote about riding the roller coaster in relation to mindfulness.
4. How does the information in this chapter affect you personally? What insights did you have about yourself and the stress that you experience?

ACTIVITY 2 - RELAXATION EXERCISE - FLOWING COMFORT

Objectives: The purpose of this activity is to allow you to practice deep relaxation on your own using the DVD relaxation exercise titled Flowing Comfort.

Materials needed:
You will need your own copy of the Stress Relief DVD and Handout 7:1 called DVD Relaxation Exercise - Flowing Comfort.

Instructions: Follow the directions on Handout 7:1.

Handout 7:1 DVD Relaxation Exercise
Flowing Comfort

The DVD homework assignment for this week is the second exercise on the Stress Relief DVD called "Flowing Comfort."

Practice doing this exercise at least two (2) times according to the instructions on the DVD. One of those times, do it immediately before you fall asleep at night. Make it the last thing you do before you close your eyes to fall asleep.

Do it at times when you will not be disturbed. It lasts approximately 19 minutes.

In a *typed* format, respond to the following items:

1. How you felt before the exercise
2. Your experience during the exercise
3. How you felt immediately following the exercise
4. How you felt long after completing the exercise, or how you slept and awakened the following morning

On your typed paper, **thoroughly** respond to each of these items referring to the two times that you did them at home, *and* the time that you did it in class. Describe primarily how you were feeling in relation to your stress levels.

Follow this general outline with your description:

Afternoon:
- Before
- During
- Immediately after
- Long after

Right before bed:
- Before
- How quickly you fell asleep
- How you slept
- How refreshed you felt in the morning
- How this differed from a typical night's sleep

Classroom experience:
- Before
- During
- Immediately after
- Long after

ACTIVITY 3 – MEDITATIVE EXERCISE: INTERNAL MINDFULNESS - THOUGHT WATCHING

Objectives: The purpose of this activity is to allow you to experience mindful meditation as it is described in the text.

Materials needed:
A quiet room, dim lighting if possible.

Duration of Activity: 10-12 minutes

Description of Activity: Close your eyes and sit quietly in your chair. As you do this, go inside your mind and simply watch your thoughts as they come and go. Be present with the thoughts, allowing them to enter and leave. Just observe. If your mind wanders or gets caught up in your thoughts, simply bring your awareness back to being an observer of all of your mental chatter as it occurs to you to do so.

After about 10 minutes of this practice, return to eyes open and fully alert.

Some ideas to consider as you practice thought watching:
- You aren't your thoughts; you are the one having the thoughts.
- When you do this on your own, have a notebook by your side because intuition happens in the spaces between thoughts.
- It is our distracting mind chatter that prevents a clear channel to intuition.

Eugene Pascal wrote, "All of man's troubles stem from his inability to sit quietly in a room alone."

To connect to our souls and discover *a spiritual solution to all of our problems,* we can learn to be still and "sit quietly in a room alone." Only in the stillness can we hear our intuition. This type of meditation is a powerful way to become still.

ACTIVITY 4 – MINDFUL HEARING AND TOUCH

Objectives: The purpose of this activity is to allow you to experience mindfulness through the senses of hearing and touch.

Materials needed:
For this activity you will need a blindfold, an open area where there are a variety of obstacles such as a children's playground, and Handout 7:2 - Mindful Touch and Hearing.

Duration of Activity: At least 25-30 minutes or as long as you would like to do it.

Description of Activity:
Once you have found an ideal place with lots of safe obstacles, put on your blindfold. It is a good idea to have someone watch you as you do this to make sure you stay safe. In this safe place you do nothing but walk around and touch and hear everything you can.

Spend 30 minutes getting totally involved with the experience. Focus on discovery. Pretend you are a curious blind child exploring some interesting place for the first time.

Once you are finished, process the experience. Sense what you noticed while you were focusing on the events. Thoughts of fears of future events weren't present to you because you were too focused on your present experience.

Use Handout 7:2 - Mindful Touch and Hearing to help you describe your experience of being mindful using your senses of hearing and touch.

Handout 7:2 - Mindful Touch and Hearing

Describe your experience of eliminating your eyesight and focusing on being mindful using your senses of hearing and touch. Include your thoughts and feelings about what you discovered, how your perceptions changed as the exercise continued, and what you noticed about your senses. Also discuss what you noticed about your stress levels as you participated in this activity.

ACTIVITY 5 - MINDFUL EATING

Objectives: The purpose of this activity is to allow you to experience mindfulness using your sense of taste

Materials needed:
Handout 7:3 - Mindful Eating

Description of Activity: Follow the directions on Handout 7:3 - Mindful Eating. Be aware that you are to go eat somewhere completely by yourself and without any other activity going on. The whole focus of this exercise is to eat food mindfully.

Be sure to give yourself sufficient time to complete this activity. Do it at a time when you can easily fit this activity into your schedule for a sufficient amount of time.

When you are finished with the exercise, type your thoughts about this activity using the instructions provided in the handout.

Handout 7:3 - Mindful Eating

The typical way of eating is to thoughtlessly shove food into our mouths, take a few brief chews of that food, and send the only-partly-chewed food down to the stomach to work overtime on those portions that have hardly been broken down. It's no wonder we get tired after a meal. This exercise breaks us out of that mode of eating.

For this assignment, you will go, **by yourself**, to a place that serves food that you love. It doesn't matter what kind of food or what kind of restaurant that you choose. It only matters that you are by yourself and that the food appeals to you.

You are going to experience this food mindfully. This means you will focus on the experience of eating your food to the exclusion of everything else. You will deliberately chew your food focusing on the taste of each bite as it combines with your saliva, touches parts of your tongue to explode with taste, and gets broken down bite by bite.

You will focus on the joy and wonder of allowing this food to literally become a part of you. Tune in to all the smells and varieties of tastes that you encounter.

If you do this in a hurry because you have seemingly more important things to do, you have failed. Remember, when we are acting mindfully, no moment has more importance than any other. When you are finished, go immediately to your computer and thoroughly write about your experience of mindful eating. Be sure to put your name on your paper and turn it in according to instructions.

ACTIVITY 6 - FULL MINDFULNESS ACTIVITY

Objectives: The purpose of this activity is to allow you to experience mindfulness using your ability to observe with all your senses.

Materials needed:
Handout 7:4 - Full Mindfulness Activity, lots of paper and a pen.

Description of Activity: Follow the instructions listed on the handout. Be sure to go somewhere completely by yourself and, for about an hour, do nothing but observe. During this exercise avoid, as much as possible, talking with anyone.

This activity can be done virtually anywhere but somewhere outdoors oftentimes is more appealing.

When you are finished, process your experience by answering the questions at the end of the handout.

Handout 7:4 - Full Mindfulness Activity

Keeping in mind the principles from chapter 7 and your class discussion on mindfulness this assignment invites you to practice being fully mindful.

During this activity, you are going to go somewhere **completely by yourself.** You will NOT talk to anyone. NO SPEAKING ALLOWED!

For a minimum of one hour, you will focus on the present moment to the exclusion of all past, future & elsewhere thoughts (imaginations, illusions, hallucinations). You will move through each of your senses, including your internal ones, and describe what shows up, as you show up for it. You will turn off your critical mind, the one that makes judgments about everything. You will simply get in touch with your experience of what is (happening).

You will begin each moment with the simple statement, "I am noticing …" as you discover all the things that present themselves to you. Use all your senses to experience mindfully what has always been *here and now* but you may have missed because your thoughts were focused on some other time and somewhere else. Don't look *for* anything - just look. On your paper, write down the things that you observe with each of your senses. Also write down the thoughts that you notice you are having during this time. If you find yourself getting bored or resisting the process, stop, look, notice what shows up, and then continue.

At the top of your page write "I AM NOTICING …" just once, then for an hour finish the sentence over and over based on what your senses bring to you.

When you are finished, summarize your experience on a separate piece of paper according to these items:

1. What were some of the main things that you observed, especially those things you wouldn't normally notice?
2. What did you notice about your thoughts?
3. What did you notice about your feelings?
4. What insights did you gain about yourself and about mindfulness as you were practicing being mindful?
5. What did you notice about your stress levels as you immersed yourself fully in your experience?

RELATED WEBSITES

Mindfulness
Excellent article an the application of mindfulness by Ernest M. Shaw, MD.
http://www.healthology.com/focus_article.asp?f=alt_medicine&c=alt_mindfulness

Mindfulness—wik.ed
Excellent overview of mindfulness
http://wik.ed.uiuc.edu/index.php/Mindfulness

Mindfulness (Sati)
Another excellent writing on mindfulness
http://www.vipassana.com/meditation/mindfulness_in_plain_english_15.php

CHAPTER 8
MANAGING EMOTIONS

CHAPTER OUTLINE

Use this outline to take notes as you read the chapter in the text and/or as your instructor lectures in class.

I. **MANAGING EMOTIONS**
    A. The ability to experience a wide range of emotions is part of what makes us uniquely human and keeps life interesting.
        1. We all get angry.
        2. We all get scared.
        3. We all feel guilt and worry.
        4. How boring life would be if we never experienced the ups and downs of our emotions.
        5. Like most things in life, there is a healthy balance for optimal well-being.
            a) Chronic guilt and worry, fear that prevents us from living life fully, and an attitude of hostility and anger are negative and stress-producing.

II. **THE PHYSIOLOGY OF EMOTIONS**
    A. Certain emotions can make you more susceptible to stress and disease.
        1. Worry, guilt, fear, anger and other strong emotions can activate the stress response.
            a) The emotions of fear and anger have been linked to the fight-or-flight response where they can serve a protective function.
                (1) Fear relates to "flight" where we see that sometimes running from or escaping from a potentially dangerous situation can protect us.
                (2) Anger relates to "fight" where the stress response is useful not to run away, but to confront and resist that which is perceived as dangerous.
        2. As many as half of all patients who visit physicians have physical symptoms that are directly caused by emotions.
            (1) Some research findings even put that figure as high as 90 to 95 percent.

III. **GUILT AND WORRY**
    A. **Guilt** is the conscious preoccupation with undesirable past thoughts and behaviors.
        1. Guilt is an expression of self-anger detected by internal dialogue that includes self-talk such as "I should have…"
    B. **Worry** is the conscious preoccupation with events yet to come.
        1. Worry is a state in which we dwell on something so much it causes us to become apprehensive.
    C. Guidelines to help you manage worry.
        1. Most things we worry about are out of our control.
        2. Worry is not the same as caring.
        3. Worry is not the same thing as planning.
        4. Most worries never happen.
        5. Write it down.
        6. Practice mindfulness
        7. Remember, worry is a habit.
    D. Letting go of guilt
        1. When we reflect on our actions and learn from them, we learn important lessons.
        2. Getting buried in the guilt of our past mistakes is not productive and only adds to our stress.
        3. To let go of guilt we need to ask ourselves a couple questions.
            a) What can I do to make it right?
            b) What lessons can I learn that will enable this experience to add value to my

life and the lives of others?

IV. FEAR

A. **Fear** is a state of escalated worry and apprehension.

B. Fear usually involves a focus on the future.

C. We create in our mind thoughts that something in our future, some event or experience, is going to involve pain, danger, or discomfort and therefore is to be avoided.

D. Types of fear (See Table 8.1)

    1. Fear of change - like moving to a new city or a breakup with a boyfriend or girlfriend.

    2. Fear of pain or other bodily suffering - like the fear we feel when we think about going to the dentist or getting a shot.

    3. Fear of failure - like not being selected for the track team or not being accepted into graduate school.

    4. Fear of punishment - like the fear that prevents people from doing things that are against the law.

    5. Fear of something - like snakes or spiders or of being in a car accident or being mugged.

    6. Fear of the unknown - like going away to school or being afraid of people who are different than you.

    7. Fear of death - the biggest unknown of them all.

E. Fear can paralyze and incapacitate you and can stop you from going after your desires.

F. There is a general desire among humans to grow, to develop, to serve, and to enjoy.

G. We have a natural tendency to want to expand, to become more of who we are.

H. In contrast to our innate need to grow and expand is the tendency to gravitate toward our comfort zones.

    1. A **comfort zone** is any place, situation, relationship or experience where we do not feel any threat. It is usually a known place or situation where we feel safe and in control.

I. For growth to happen, we must leave our comfort zones and move out into our **discomfort zones.**

    1. This growth takes effort. Included in this effort is usually overcoming or dealing with some type of fear.

    2. We feel that there might be pain or discomfort of some kind in our discomfort zones.

        a) The reality is that when we move out into the discomfort zone, we are rarely hurt, in the true sense where physical pain is involved.

        b) Consider the example of speaking in public.

        c) At no time during the process of preparing or during the speech is real pain inflicted on the speaker.

    3. Anytime we find ourselves afraid of something, we can mentally examine each step prior to the event and the event itself, and remove any unreal pain.

        a) By realizing that there is no real pain except that which we create in our own minds, we can choose to think differently about it.

V. PUTTING IT TOGETHER

A. Four principles for managing fear can shape our understanding of fear and guide us in taking control of our choices.

    1. Fear can motivate positive action.

    2. Nothing in the world is inherently frightening.

    3. Fear is learned

    4. With practice and experience we learn to overcome our fears.

B. Strategy for overcoming fear

    1. First, admit you are afraid.

    2. Next, confront your fear.

    3. Do whatever it is that you are so afraid of at least three times.

    4. As you confront your fear, call it something else - excitement or a challenge, for example.

VI. THE FEAR-FAITH CONNECTION

A. The more we believe that our lives are about something, that things happen for a reason, and that we are meant to benefit from the experience of our journey, the more courageous and less fearful we are when confronted with difficult situations.

B. The more we are guided by fear, the weaker our faith; the stronger our faith, the less we fear.

    1. Not just faith related to your beliefs in a higher power, but also about the faith you have in yourself and your abilities.

C. You will never overcome all your fears, but you can conquer the fears that prevent you from living your life to the fullest.

D. The more you associate pleasure and positive feelings with risking, the more you will be inclined to risk again.

VII. ANGER

A. **Anger** is a powerful emotion based on wanting something, not getting it, and feeling frustrated.

B. Anger comes in many forms including abuse, ridicule, physical violence, temper tantrums, sarcasm, and even the silent treatment.

C. Anger and Hostility

    1. Hostility and anger are not interchangeable terms even though they are frequently used that way.

        a) Anger is considered a temporary emotion, usually in response to a specific event.

        b) **Hostility** is an attitude motivated by hatefulness and animosity.

        c) Hostility is especially dangerous for heart health and may be a good predictor of heart attacks.

        d) Anger and hostility appear to have a dampening effect on the body's immune system.

        e) People who are hostile tend to be involved in abuse and problems with marriage, higher levels of stress, less job satisfaction, and more problems in working relationships.

D. Effects of anger

    1. The effects of anger are very much like the harmful effects of chronic stress.

        a) Studies are showing that the harmful effects of anger may even be more dangerous to our health than the stress response.

E. Sources of anger

    1. There are many reasons people become angry, and anger has many sources.

F. Breaking the rules

    1. Ultimately anger is always a response to an event that we feel didn't go as we wanted it to go.

        a) Someone has broken one of our rules - our beliefs about how things should be.

    2. The event, of itself, does not make us angry any more than events can make us feel stressed, bored, or any other emotion.

        a) The way we construct the event mentally in our minds, what it means to us, determines whether or not we will become angry.

        b) We can immediately defuse any bout of anger simply by reexamining our rule and being aware that it is our rule and not the event itself that is causing us to choose anger.

    3. If we notice ourselves feeling that something ought to be different than it is and we are in a position to make positive changes, we can channel our anger into productive action.

G. Expressing anger

1. Expressing anger is healthy, but how you express that anger may be even more important to your well-being.
    a) So "venting" may make you feel better, but only for the moment.
H. Anger Blockers
    1. See the list following Anger Blockers for ideas to help prevent anger.

VIII.   CONCLUSION
A. The ability to experience a wide range of emotions is part of what makes us human and keeps life interesting.
B. The challenge is in taking responsibility to control the negative emotions that can decrease quality of life.
    1. Long-term emotions like fear, worry, and anger can affect health and longevity in much the same way as long-term stress.
C. Take control of your emotions so they don't take control of you.

LEARNING ACTIVITIES

ACTIVITY 1 - JOURNALING

Objective: The purpose of this activity is to encourage critical thinking and honest personal reflection on topics relating to the chapter content. Explore personal thoughts, feelings, values, and behaviors as you selectively incorporate stress management knowledge and behaviors into your plan for improved health through better stress management.

Instructions: You will find journaling questions in each chapter of your Activities Manual. These questions relate specifically to the chapter content. Moving your thoughts from your mind to the paper is a powerful strategy for relieving stress and for increasing awareness of your thoughts, feelings and behaviors. Your course instructor can provide further guidance on how to complete this activity.

Complete the following journaling questions. Select the questions that have the most relevance for you.

1. Think about the last time you were really angry about something. Think about the rule that you constructed that was the reason for the emotion of anger. What is a different way of thinking about the event that puts you in control of your anger?
2. Describe how you feel about the notion that life is about growing, overcoming our fears, and moving outside of our comfort zones.
3. Think of a time when you felt like you were outside of your comfort zone. Reflect on this experience in relation to the point made in the chapter that the discomfort is created by your thoughts about the situation and not the situation itself. In other words, why is there no real discomfort in our discomfort zone?
4. In this chapter we learn that the only real way to overcome our fears is by dealing directly with whatever we fear. Think of a time when this was the case for you. How does this help you as you think of other fears that get in the way of you getting what you want?
5. According to the information in this chapter, the only reason why you ever get angry at anyone or anything is because one of your rules has been broken. The anger isn't about what someone else did, but because of your rule. How does this idea change your thinking about the times you have gotten angry at people or situations?
6. How does the information in this chapter affect you personally? What insights did you have about yourself and the stress that you experience?

ACTIVITY 2 - FEEL THE FEAR - GO FOR IT ANYWAY

Objectives: The purpose of this activity is to allow you to participate in an activity that is well outside of your comfort zones.

Materials needed:
Handout 8:1 – Feel the Fear - Go for it Anyway
Handout 8:2 – Supporting Thoughts on Fear

Description of Activity: Review the instructions on the "Feel the Fear" handout. Take a hard look at what you really fear and then go for it!

Handout 8:1 - Feel the Fear and Do It Anyway

Think of something that you are quite nervous or fearful of doing. Not just something with a tiny bit of fear, but that big one you know should be done, but you have been avoiding for quite a while because your fears of what might or might not happen are stopping you. It is something that is definitely outside of your comfort zones.

Your assignment is to break through your fear and take a risk. Do that thing that you have feared. Don't just go through the motions, do the whole thing. If it doesn't cause you to leave your comfort zone, that wasn't the thing you fear. Decide on something that causes you to want to back off just from the thought of it.

Begin this activity by describing (using your word processor) the thing you fear doing. Relate your thoughts and feelings about why it seems to be fearful for you.

After you have completed the assignment describe your experience from beginning to end of going for it and doing the thing you really feared. Also, describe any insights you gained about that particular fear and your thoughts about it. Describe any insights you have gained about your own fears in general.

Remember Shakespeare's famous line on fear: "Our doubts are traitors and cause us to lose the good we oft might win for fearing to attempt."

Examples of students' fear from previous classes:

- Ask somebody out on a date
- Quit a job
- Confront someone
- Forgive someone
- Interview for a job
- Speak in a public meeting
- Go rock climbing (fear of heights)
- Change majors
- Mend a broken relationship
- Tell someone who you have avoided that you love him or her
- Visit someone you don't know very well but would like to and get to know him or her better

You may have already done something previously that you felt was fearful. That's great! For this assignment do something else.

You may ask what this has to do with stress management and why you are being asked to do something that only increases your stress levels. Breaking through fears and taking risks is like a muscle. The more you do it, the more easy doing fearful things becomes in the future, and the less stressful they seem. When you are no longer stopped by your fears, you have gained a huge upper hand on stress. Get hooked on this idea and there is no limit to what you can become and attain! So go for it!

Handout 8:2 - Supporting Thoughts on Fear

Principles of Managing Fear and Taking Risks
1. Fear is a belief that an outcome will include some pain or discomfort
   a. This belief stops us from moving forward toward an outcome
2. Nothing in the world is inherently fearful
3. All Fear is learned
4. There is no pain in our discomfort zone except what we create
5. We must adopt the feeling of assurance that we can handle it
6. Disassociate the pain with the steps and the outcome
   a. Determine where the pain is - assess the reality
7. The only way to overcome fear is through it
8. The only way to get better at handling fear is by practice

Life is about growth. Growth involves giving up something without knowing for certain if the next step will be any better. If this weren't the case, we would call it "sure thing taking" rather than risk taking.

Helen Keller's words on Risking & Security:
Security is mostly a superstition. It does not exist in nature, nor do the children of men as a whole experience it. Avoiding danger is no safer in the long run than outright exposure. Life is either a daring adventure or nothing.

Any risk that is important for growth will continually reappear until it is settled.

The knowledge that you can handle anything that comes your way is the key to allowing yourself to take risks. If you knew you could handle anything that came your way, what would you possibly have to fear? Answer: Nothing.

All you have to do to diminish your fear is develop more trust in your ability to handle whatever comes your way.
        Why do we sense we can't handle stuff?
                An overriding "Be careful" mentality
                It isn't too important to know all the reasons for our fears.
        Whatever happens in any situation, I can handle it.
                How do I know? My history!
Underlying all of our fears is a lack of trust in ourselves.
        What we must remember is we CAN handle it.

Self affirming statements on fear:
1) The fear will never go away as long as I continue to grow
   a) Relax into the possibility that this is the purpose of living
2) The only way to get rid of the fear of doing something is to go out and Do It.
3) The only way to feel better about myself is to go out ... and do it.
   a) The *doing it* comes before the *feeling better* part
4) Not only am I going to experience fear whenever I'm on unfamiliar territory, but so is everyone else.
   a) Fear isn't a signal to retreat, but a green light to move ahead.
5) Pushing through fear is less frightening than living with the underlying fear that comes with a feeling of helplessness.
The challenges we face are what makes us grow - that's the real outcome.
        Security is not having things, it's handling things.

Before making a decision:
1. Focus on the no-lose model*
2. Do your homework. No false starts - only steps along the way
3. Establish your priorities

4. Trust your impulses
5. Lighten up - don't take things so seriously

*no-lose model: In the moment of decision, a no-lose possibility looks at every decision, every alternative as being filled with opportunities - regardless of the outcome. *"It's all an adventure, no matter which way I turn."* The outcome can be reduced to irrelevance. In the no lose model, it is impossible to make a mistake. Mistakes must be seen in a new light. Consider the inventor who discovers 900 ways not to reach an outcome or the baseball batter who only hits 3 out of 10 times.

After making a decision:
1. Throw away your picture - Don't focus on "the way it is supposed to be."
2. Accept total responsibility for your decisions
3. Don't protect, correct - if it isn't working, change.
> A plane flight to Hawaii is off course 90% of the time. Always correcting.
> Clues for when to correct: confusion and dissatisfaction

Keep in mind: few things really matter - including what other people think. We must eliminate the "what will they think" mentality.

Magic Duo - commit 100% to what you are doing
> Act as if you and what you are doing matters - you count!

Just say "yes" - stop resisting what is
> Saying no means to operate as a victim, to resist, blocking the flow
> Opportunities open up to "yes."
> Saying yes doesn't mean giving up. It means getting up and acting on your belief that you can create meaning and purpose in whatever life gives you.

Fear involves a sensation of losing something. Paradoxically, we only retain, keep, what we give away. And if we want more of something, we get that by giving it. When we hang on to things, we live in lack. When we give, we live in abundance.

Your life is more than one component. If you lose that one component (a relationship, for example), you are left with nothing - empty. Fill life up with all roles and commit to live 100% in each role, when you are in it (at work, with a spouse, playing with kids). If you don't feel it, act "as if" you are fully committed to it. Show up and be fully present.

You must become what you want to attract (the truth is, there is no other reality - you attract what you are.

When you are aware of the fact that "you have," you give. When you are a giver, you have nothing to fear.

> Partially based on Susan Jeffers' book, "Feel the Fear and Do It Anyway"[1]

---

[1] Jeffers, S. (1987). Feel the fear and do it anyway. New York: Ballantine Books.

ACTIVITY 3- BOX YOUR EMOTIONS

Objective: The purpose of this activity is to assist you in taking control of your emotions by differentiating between what is in your control and what is not.

Instructions: Complete Handout 8:3 - Box Your Emotions. An example is provided below.

BOX YOUR EMOTIONS

IMPORTANT & CONTROLLABLE	NOT IMPORTANT & CONTROLLABLE
• *I'm frustrated* when phone calls disrupt our evening meal. • *I'm worried* that my credit card debt is too large. • *I'm disgusted* with myself for not getting more exercise.	• *I really hate it* when my husband leaves the toilet seat up. • *I'm angry* when the newspaper delivery girl throws the paper in the bushes.
IMPORTANT & NOT CONTROLLABLE	**NOT IMPORTANT & NOT CONTROLLABLE**
• *I'm worried* that my dad will die from lung cancer. • *I'm angry* that it rained on my wedding.	• *I'm afraid* of getting older. • *It feel so mad* when it rains after I wash my car.

Handout 8:3 - Box Your Emotions

Instructions: Over the next two to three days, examine the stresses in your life. Think about the emotions associated with both the big and little stresses that occur day in and day out. For instance, what makes you angry, worried, frustrated, fearful or depressed? Just jot down the stress-producing emotion and what causes it. For example, you're list might include such things as:

- I'm furious that my teacher scheduled a big test on the day we get back from spring break.
- I'm sad that my best friend is transferring to another school.
- I'm afraid that my credit card debt is growing out of control.

Once you have made a list of the emotions you are experiencing, go back to your list and decide in which box each stressor would best fit.

IMPORTANT & CONTROLLABLE	*NOT* IMPORTANT & CONTROLLABLE
IMPORTANT & *NOT* CONTROLLABLE	***NOT* IMPORTANT & *NOT* CONTROLLABLE**

Focus on the emotions and activities associated with events that are not in your control. What can you do to prevent negative, stressful emotions related to things that are not in your control?

ACTIVITY 4 – DEALING WITH ANGER – IT'S ALL ABOUT YOUR RULES

Objectives: The purpose of this activity is to invite you to see the real reason why you get angry at anything.

Description of Activity: Review the section in chapter 8 of your textbook on anger. Remember that the real reason why you find yourself getting angry is not because of the situation in your environment, but rather, the rules you've made about the situation that have been broken—either by you or by someone or something else.

Think about a situation in which you noticed yourself getting upset, angry, or mad at someone or something that happened. Write it down here:

Now think about the rule that you have made about the situation that was broken. Remember that a rule is a belief you've made up about how something ought to be or how someone ought to act. The rule behind your anger that was broken was:

As always, your rule being broken, and not the situation or person involved, was what caused you to have feelings of anger.

RELATED WEBSITES

Know No Fear
Thoughts on overcoming fear by Rick Beneteau
http://faculty.weber.edu/molpin/healthclasses/1110/nofear.htm

Basic Emotions
Learn to recognize emotions at increasing levels of detail. If you can see the emotion, then you can respond appropriately to it.
http://changingminds.org/explanations/emotions/basic%20emotions.htm

Ditch the Comfort Zone
Interesting thoughts on Comfort Zones by Neal Burgis, Ph.D.
http://www.jewishaz.com/jewishnews/041029/ditch.shtml

CHAPTER 9
THE IMPORTANCE OF VALUES

CHAPTER OUTLINE
Use this outline to take notes as you read the chapter in the text and/or as your instructor lectures in class.

I. **UNDERSTANDING YOUR VALUES**
    A. A **value** can be defined as a belief upon which one acts by preference.
        1. Values guide our actions and give direction and meaning to one's life.
        2. Decision-making comes down to how we value those things on which we are deciding.
            a) When you know what is most important to you, making the best decision is much easier.
            b) When you are unclear about what you value most, making the best decision is more difficult.
                (1) The result is inner conflict and stress.
        3. Knowing our values and then learning to live by them is one of the most powerful ways to gain inner peace and decrease stress.
            a) Not only does this apply to the bigger life decisions, but our everyday choices as well.
    B. Discovering our values
        1. **Dharma** is a principle that includes the idea that every person who has ever lived is a specific piece of an enormous puzzle of several billion pieces (one for each person).
            a) Your personal piece of this gigantic puzzle is a specific size and shape and fits correctly in only one precise place in this puzzle.
        2. Dharma teaches us that when you find your place in the puzzle, you find satisfaction in life; you feel fulfilled, happy, and worthwhile.
        3. The natural consequences are inner peace, wisdom, and happiness.
            a) We feel fulfilled and satisfied with ourselves and the direction in which our life is going when we are certain about who we are.
    C. **Cognitive dissonance** relates to situations where our behavior is inconsistent with our beliefs, values or self-image.
        1. Most people do not pay much attention to their values until they find themselves in a situation where they feel in conflict with their values.
            a) The tension created by the dissonance causes you to look more closely at your values and make a direct decision based on them.

II. **THE NIAGARA SYNDROME**
    A. When we don't discover our guiding principles we float toward what Anthony Robbins calls the **Niagara Syndrome**.
        1. We hit a disaster waiting to happen in a boat with no oars.
        2. We are going to experience some kind of fall.
    B. Stephen Covey relates a similar analogy of the person who spends his entire life climbing the ladder of success only to realize, when he arrives at the top, his ladder is leaning against the wrong wall.

III. **SOURCE OF VALUES**
    A. We tend to base our values on several sources, namely, our **culture**, our parental and familial influences, our teachers, friends, and other environmental influences such as television, the Internet and a host of other media outlets.

IV. **THE DYNAMIC QUALITY OF VALUES**
    A. A personal value system is not static.
        1. When we are young, our values mirror those of our parents or teachers.
        2. As we move through adolescence and young adulthood, we may challenge the

values we learned as a child and develop more personal values resulting from a mixture of what we learned from our parents and what we have chosen to embrace from our culture.

V. **VALUES WITHIN CULTURES**
    A. Certain values are predominant in our culture:
        1. Personal Achievement and Success
        2. Activity and Work
        3. Moral Orientation
        4. Efficiency and Practicality
        5. Progress
        6. Material Comfort
        7. Personal Freedom and Individualism
        8. External Conformity
        9. Science and Rationality

VI. **ACQUIRING VALUES**
    A. **Values acquisition** is the conscious assumption of a new value.
    B. There are seven steps for values acquisition:
        1. Step 1: The value is chosen freely.
        2. Step 2: The value is chosen from among alternatives.
        3. Step 3: The value is chosen after careful consideration of each alternative.
        4. Step 4: The value is prized and cherished.
        5. Step 5: The value is publicly affirmed.
        6. Step 6: The value is acted upon.
        7. Step 7: The value is part of a pattern of repeated action (value is incorporated into the individual's lifestyle).

VII. **BELIEFS ABOUT VALUES**
    A. To make positive change in the direction of our own true path, there are several beliefs that we must firmly maintain in our minds to support us as we begin our journey.
        1. We must first believe that we are capable of changing our thoughts and actions.
        2. We must also have the belief that if we are going to create long-term change in our lives, that we are responsible.
        3. We must have the belief that if we set our sites in a new direction, and then move confidently in that direction, we will successfully arrive near the place we wanted to go.
        4. We must be certain that our values determine our actions and behaviors.

VIII. **TYPES OF VALUES**
    A. **Instrumental values** consist, primarily, of personal characteristics and character traits.
        1. Instrumental values involve ways of being that help us arrive at terminal values.
        2. Instrumental values help get us to our terminal values.
    B. **Terminal values** are those outcomes that we work toward or we believe are most important and desirable.
        1. Terminal values are end states of feeling; they are the emotional state that you prefer experiencing.
        2. Terminal values make our life fulfilling and worthwhile.

IX. **VALUES CLARIFICATION**
    A. **Values clarification**, the process of helping you clarify and apply what you truly value, is very helpful for reducing the stress that comes from making choices that are inconsistent with your values.
        1. Values clarification is a cognitive process that helps close the gap between what an individual says and actually does.

X. **CREATING YOUR PERSONAL CONSTITUTION**
    A. Step 1 - Identify your values
        1. Follow the activities in this section of the book.

    B. Step 2 - Prioritize your values
        1. Take your list of values and prioritize them in order of importance to you.
        2. Knowing the order of your highest values is important in decision making.
        3. Ask yourself these questions:
            a) What would be the single most important value that would propel you toward living your life the most fully?
            b) What would be the next most important value that you could integrate into your life that would have the greatest positive affect?

    C. Step 3 - Write a clarifying paragraph for your values in the form of an **affirmation**.
        1. Write your affirmation as a *positive statement*.
        2. Write your clarifying affirmations as *"I" messages*.
        3. Write your clarifying paragraph in the *present tense* as if it is currently happening.

    D. After many months of very hard work, the founding fathers of our country created the United States Constitution.
        1. This document of national values guides the creation of all laws that are made in every court of law in the entire country.
        2. Similarly, on a personal level, our own "personal constitution" can be our inner guide to all decisions that we make during our lifetime.

XI. CONCLUSION
    A. A ship without a rudder wanders aimlessly in the sea.
    B. Similarly, if we don't know why we are here and what is most important to us, we spend a lot of time in our lives wondering and wandering aimlessly.
        1. Values clarification and acquisition puts the rudder in the water and helps us move in the direction that is best for each of us on a personal level.
    C. The goal of values clarification is to facilitate self-understanding.
        1. Your values become the basis for every decision that you make.

<u>LEARNING ACTIVITIES</u>

ACTIVITY 1 - JOURNALING

Objective: The purpose of this activity is to encourage critical thinking and honest personal reflection on topics relating to the chapter content. Explore personal thoughts, feelings, values, and behaviors as you selectively incorporate stress management knowledge and behaviors into your plan for improved health through better stress management.

Instructions: You will find journaling questions in each chapter of your Activities Manual. These questions relate specifically to the chapter content. Moving your thoughts from your mind to the paper is a powerful strategy for relieving stress and for increasing awareness of your thoughts, feelings and behaviors. Your course instructor can provide further guidance on how to complete this activity.

Complete the following journaling questions. Select the questions that have the most relevance for you.

1. Think about your personal constitution, including your prioritized values and clarifying paragraphs. How do you feel this process can help you with important decisions that you will be making in the future?
2. Explain how your life is like a piece in a giant jigsaw puzzle and why it is important to find your place.
3. Put in your own words your understanding of the Niagara Syndrome.
4. Explain the natural consequences of living (how you spend your time), and not living, according to your own values.
5. Think of a situation in which you were acutely aware of an internal conflict between your values and your actions. How did this conflict result in an increase in your stress?
6. Look at the tables of Instrumental and Terminal Values. Clarify the main difference between the two and then write one instrumental and one terminal value that you have that are not on these lists.
7. Explain what Ben Franklin realized was the key to his success and how you think that contributed to his success as a self-realized individual and a founding father of our country.
8. Read through the predominant American values found in Box 9-1. Do you agree that these are predominant values? Analyze each value. We sometimes find that our values are so deeply ingrained that we have trouble seeing alternatives. How do you think these values might contribute to stress in society. Create an alternative value to each of those listed. Investigate and share examples demonstrating cultures that place higher value on some of these alternatives.
9. How does the information in this chapter affect you personally? What insights did you have about yourself and the stress that you experience?

ACTIVITY 2 - CLARIFYING MY GOVERNING VALUES

Objectives: The purpose of this activity is to help you discover and prioritize your governing values

Materials needed:
Handout 9:1 - Identifying and Prioritizing My Governing Values
Handout 9:2 - Making a clarifying statement for each of your values

Description of Activity: This activity should follow a classroom discussion on the content of chapter 9.

Begin with the two handouts, but don't write anything on them until later.

You will need someone to help you with this step. Find a quiet place where you can close your eyes while remaining seated. Ask someone to slowly read the script from chapter 9 titled "Your Funeral."

Once you are finished with this script, begin to list on the left side of the handout titled *Identifying and Prioritizing My Governing Values* each of your own values, in no particular order, according to your impressions from the Your Funeral script. Also, refer to the list of Instrumental and Terminal Values in Chapter 9. Take as much time as you need to think of all of those values that you feel apply to you.

Next, move to the right column of the same page and, with the values you have listed on the left side, prioritize or rank them according to the worth the values have to you. Your top value is written on the top line.

Consider this question "If I were to really design my own life, if I were going to create a set of values that will shape the ultimate destiny I desire, what would they need to be and in what order?" Take some time to rearrange and add to your list with this question in mind.

The next step of this process is to take each one of your values and write a clarifying statement/affirmation about it. Practice doing this on the second handout titled *"Making a clarifying statement for each of your values."* Begin with the first value you listed on the right side of the handout. Consider the following guidelines from Chapter 9 as you write them:
- Write your affirmation as a *positive statement*.
- Write your clarifying affirmations as *"I" messages*
- Write your clarifying paragraph in the *present tense* as if it is currently happening.

Follow the examples and additional details outlined in Chapter 9.

Handout 9:1 –Identifying and Prioritizing My Governing Values

What matters most to me in life? What is most important to me and what do I value the most? What value, idea or principle has such great worth that I would dedicate my life to be able to live that value?

In your text there are two activities that can help you with this process. In the left column below, list all the values that came to mind as you thought of your own funeral as well as the lists of Instrumental and Terminal. Do not list them in any order, but simply write down all those values that seem to be worthwhile to you.

Next, consider each of the values you wrote in the first column and in the right column rank them according to their worth to you. As you are doing this, You may want to consider the following question "If I were to really design my own life, if I were going to create a set of values that shape the ultimate destiny I desired, what would they need to be and in what order?"

	Values (in no particular order)		Values (in order of priority)
1		1	
2		2	
3		3	
4		4	
5		5	
6		6	
7		7	
8		8	
9		9	
10		10	
11		11	
12		12	

Don't be concerned about the number of values you feel that you have. If you have more than the number of lines in this table, turn over the page and continue there.

Handout 9:2 – Making a Clarifying Statement for Each of Your Values

Write a clarifying statement for each value. Answer the question for yourself, what does this value really mean to you?" If you were living that value perfectly, what would your behavior be like? Write as an affirmation. These are positive statement describing something as if it has already occurred. These can be as short as one line or as long as a paragraph.

Value #1 _____

Clarifying statement or paragraph

_____
_____
_____
_____
_____
_____
_____

Value #2 _____

Clarifying statement or paragraph

_____
_____
_____
_____
_____
_____
_____

This page is to be used to begin the process. The final product will be completed in a typed format using your word processor with a longer list. You will continue the same procedure for each of your values.

ACTIVITY 3 - CREATING MY PERSONAL CONSTITUTION

Objectives: The purpose of this activity is to continue the previous activity by completing a clarifying paragraph for each of your values. In the process, you are creating your own personal constitution.

Materials needed:
The two handouts you were working on for the **Clarifying My Governing Values** activity.
Chapter 9 of your textbook.

Description of Activity:
Continue with the same process adding to the values list as you have time to think about it more. Continue with the ranking process, possibly redoing it with more time to think about it. Then write a clarifying statement or paragraph for each of your values. Combine your clarifying statements into your personal constitution.

It is a good idea to take a week or two to complete this activity. Spend some time alone, preferably with some of your most inspirational books and other items that may help you think about what is most important to you. You may find it helpful to go somewhere out in nature. Really think deeply about these things. Take this assignment seriously. You are creating your own constitution upon which all of your decisions will be made.

At some point, transfer all of your work onto your computer and save a copy that you can work on in the future.

RELATED WEBSITES

Tips on Values Clarification
A key area in our self-knowledge is becoming aware of our core values. Knowing our core values or what's most important to us is extremely relevant to creating goals, setting priorities, and managing our time.
http://emoclear.com/processes/values.html

Reasoning about values - Intrinsic and instrumental values
In reasoning about values, the distinction between instrumental and intrinsic value is of fundamental importance. But first we need to understand the distinction between means and ends. This article attempts to clarify them.
http://philosophy.hku.hk/think/value/iv.php

The Wisdom Page
The Wisdom Page is a compilation of wisdom-related resources -- various on-line texts concerning wisdom, references to books about wisdom, information about organizations that promote wisdom, wise activities, and listserv groups concerned with aspects of wisdom.
http://www.cop.com/info/wisdompg.html

CHAPTER 10
SPIRITUALITY

CHAPTER OUTLINE
Use this outline to take notes as you read the chapter in the text and/or as your instructor lectures in class.

I. **SPIRITUALITY**
   A. People with a deep sense of spirituality view life differently.
      1. They have a purpose, they enjoy a sense of meaning in life, and they have a broader perspective.
      2. Decision-making comes down to how we value those things on which we are deciding.
      3. Spirituality buffers stress; people with a deep sense of spirituality are not defeated by crisis.
      4. They are able to relax their minds, elicit the relaxation response, and heal more quickly and completely.

II. **THE SPIRITUAL QUEST**
   A. With the dawn of a new century, spirituality has come to the forefront in the workplace, politics, education, and health care.
      1. People of all ages are seeking guidance on the spiritual dimension of health in the quest for fulfillment, peace and a meaningful life.
      2. Discussions of spirituality are no longer isolated to religious settings but are part of current events and daily life.
      3. We have come to acknowledge that wholeness of health incorporates body, mind, and spirit.

III. **SPIRITUALITY AND RELIGIOSITY**
   A. All humans appear to have a **spiritual dimension**, a quality that goes beyond religious affiliation, which strives for inspiration, reverence, awe, meaning, and purpose even in those who do not believe in any god.
      1. **Spirituality** is a process, a journey, the essence of life principle of a person, a belief that relates a person to the world, and a way of giving meaning to existence.
         a) It is a personal quest to find meaning and purpose in life, and a relationship or sense of connection with a higher power.
      2. **Religiosity** is a term that refers to the degree of participation in or adherence to the beliefs and practices of an organized religion.
         a) It relates to any person who accepts the tenets of, and actively participates in, an organized religion and its practices.
      3. Spirituality is a much broader concept than religiosity that also includes nonreligious beliefs and expressions.
         a) A person may be deeply spiritual yet not profess a religion.
         b) An individual may be highly religious but not spiritual.
         c) Many people find their religious beliefs and practices to be an integral aspect of their spiritual development.

IV. **RESEARCH ON SPIRITUALITY**
   A. Spiritual health is not an exact science.
   B. What is evident is that the spiritual dimension is equal to and perhaps even more important than the other dimensions of health and well-being.
      1. Spiritual health is finding its way into such common healing modalities as hypnosis, biofeedback, acupuncture, massage, and reflexology.
   C. A second challenge of spirituality research relates to the placebo effect.
      1. **Placebo** is used to describe a range of effects created by a person's belief that he or she will benefit from an intervention.
      2. It is generally believed that about 35 percent of people experience the placebo

effect.

    a) When a person believes prayers for healing will be answered, is it actually the prayer that resulted in healing or the strong belief that healing would occur that altered the mind/body response in a positive manner?

D. A review of the research literature identifies a correlation between religious activities and health outcomes.

    1. Religiosity is beneficial for mental and physical health and stress management and that it supports a healthy lifestyle.

        a) Are the health benefits from being religious due to the intervention of a higher power, or are the benefits related to variables such as social support or healthier lifestyle choices that are taught in many religions?

E. Scientific methods simply are not always adequate for exploring concepts like faith and spirituality.

    1. Great strides are being made in applying scientific research methodology to gain understanding of the impact of spiritual and religious variables on health and stress management.

    2. Still, people who turn to spirituality for comfort and healing do not need scientific studies to convince them.

V. FIVE QUALITIES OF SPIRITUAL HEALTH

A. Regardless of religious affiliation, some common qualities relate to spiritual health and stress management.

B. Five qualities of **spiritual health** cut across many religious and spiritual beliefs and have special relevance in stress management.

    1. A sense of peace, meaning, and purpose in life.

    2. Faith in God or a higher power, however you choose to define it.

    3. Feeling connected to others and seeing oneself as part of something bigger.

    4. Compassion for others.

    5. Participation in religious behaviors or meaningful spiritual rituals.

VI. MEANING AND PURPOSE

A. Without some purpose in life, we wander aimlessly and our enthusiasm for life can be lost.

B. Frankl emphasizes that while an individual may be powerless to modify his environment or even his or her physical condition, each person does have the ultimate power to fashion reactions and find *interior meaning*, even in the most difficult of circumstances.

VII. BELIEF IN A HIGHER POWER

A. A belief in a higher power is the cornerstone of every major religion and social science.

B. **Faith** is the belief in or commitment to something or someone that helps a person realize a purpose.

    1. George Sheehan credits religion with an almost unequaled power to relieve stress by providing an inner sense of calm and tranquility and a sense that no defeat is final.

    2. The result is a sense of lasting security from making connection with a higher power.

C. Important to stress management is the question of control.

    1. On one level, we have learned that we are in control of much of what happens in life.

        a) Feeling empowered and in control can be stress-relieving.

    2. On another level, it is freeing to believe that some things are simply not in our control.

        a) Believing that we can release those responsibilities that are beyond our control to a higher power relieves stress by providing a sense of tranquility and security.

    3. This faith is a partnership with a Power greater than us, a co-creatorship with God that allows us to be guided by God and yet take responsibility for our lives.

VIII. **CONNECTEDNESS**
   A. **Connectedness** is the dimension of one's being that is an integrating or unifying factor and that is manifested through unifying interconnectedness, purpose and meaning in life, innerness or inner resources and transcendence.
   B. It is the feeling of relatedness or attachment to others, a sense of relationship to all of life, a feeling of harmony with self and others, and a feeling of oneness with the universe and/or a universal element or Universal Being.
   C. Connectedness implies that there is some aspect of humanity that connects each of us with each other.
      1. The practical application of this understanding is that if you are a part of me and I am a part of you, I will be much more likely to treat you in loving and friendly ways.
         a) Functioning in more loving ways toward everyone and everything is very stress relieving.

IX. **COMPASSION FOR OTHERS**
   A. Because the spiritual dimension of health transcends the individual, it has the capacity to be a common bond between individuals.
   B. With this common bond, we are motivated to share love, warmth, and compassion with other people.
   C. Forgiveness and altruism are two important qualities of compassion that have special relevance to stress management.
      1. **Forgiveness** is the experience of psychological peace that occurs when injured people transform their grievances against others.
         a) This transformation takes place by learning to take less personal offense, to attribute less blame to the offender, and to understand the personal harm that comes from unresolved anger.
         b) People who refuse to forgive harbor resentment, anger, and bitterness.
         c) This negative attitude is harmful not only emotionally but physically, due to the release of potent stress-related hormones that cause our heart to pound, muscles to tense, and blood pressure to soar.
         d) Forgiveness is an attitude that implies that you are willing to accept responsibility for your perceptions, realizing that your perceptions are a choice and not an objective fact.
         e) When you forgive someone, you make yourself, rather than the person who hurt you, responsible for your future happiness.
      2. **Altruism** is the act of helping or giving to others without thought of self-benefit.
         a) Giving of ourselves benefits both the giver and the receiver.
         b) Many report that when they do something for someone else, without seeking any external reward, they feel inwardly happier and more content.
            (1) When we take our mind off of our own troubles and problems as we try to help someone else with theirs, our difficulties seem less significant and our stress is reduced.

X. **RELIGIOUS BEHAVIORS AND MEANINGFUL SPIRITUAL RITUALS**
   A. Evidence suggests that those who regularly prayed, read religious literature, attended church or synagogue (or other site of religious practice), and considered themselves strong and active in their religious faith reported only half the health problems as non-practicing people.
   B. Prayer is a ritual that has special relevance for stress reduction.
      1. Virtually every culture prays in one form or another, especially during times of stress and at the end of life.
      2. In prayer, people put their trust in a divine power, relax, and let go of their fears, and experience a state of great peace.
      3. Prayer has powerful beneficial physiological and psychological effects as many studies demonstrate.

C. Spending time in nature can be a profound spiritual experience.
   1. Throughout history, most religious and cultural traditions have included a connection with nature.
   2. Nature is considered by many to be the most visible manifestation of the spirit.

XI. AN ACTION PLAN
A. There are many paths to spiritual growth, but this growth starts with a single step.
   1. Begin by defining what spirituality means to you?
   2. Take a few minutes to close your eyes and reflect on some spiritual moments in your life; times when you were keenly aware of your spirituality. Describe this spiritual experience.
   3. Based on your definition of spirituality, reflect on how spirituality relates to stress in your life.
      a) Do you see a relationship between your spiritual beliefs and your values?
      b) When our actions are consistent with our values and beliefs, the outcome is balance, peace, and fulfillment.
   4. Participate in the Spiritual Wellness Assessment.

XII. WAYS TO ENHANCE SPIRITUAL HEALTH
- Prayer
- Reflection or quiet listening to one's intuition
- Communion with nature
- Enjoyment of music, drama, art, dance
- Inner dialogue with oneself or with a higher power
- Loving relationships with others
- Service to others in need
- Forgiveness
- Empathy, compassion, hope
- Laughter, joyous expressions
- Participation in a caring community - a church, a support group or any group which gives you a feeling of belonging
- Reading about spiritual growth from any source you find inspiring -the insights of others can help you formulate your own meaning and purpose in life
- Quiet time each day for prayer, meditation, or thinking - silence can be very healing and help restore a sense of balance

XIII. CONCLUSION
A. There is not one best path to spiritual health; the right way is the one that works for you.
B. Spiritual health involves a lifetime of deliberate choices and an intentional inner focus on matters of the spirit.
C. Making choices that fulfill your purpose in life will bring the ultimate stress-relievers - peace, joy, and love - into your life.
D. Spiritual health includes the quality of existence in which you are at peace with yourself and in good harmony with the environment.

<u>LEARNING ACTIVITIES</u>

ACTIVITY 1 - JOURNALING

Objective: The purpose of this activity is to encourage critical thinking and honest personal reflection on topics relating to the chapter content. Explore personal thoughts, feelings, values, and behaviors as you selectively incorporate stress management knowledge and behaviors into your plan for improved health through better stress management.

Instructions: You will find journaling questions in each chapter of your Activities Manual. These questions relate specifically to the chapter content. Moving your thoughts from your mind to the paper is a powerful strategy for relieving stress and for increasing awareness of your thoughts, feelings and behaviors. Your course instructor can provide further guidance on how to complete this activity.

Complete the following journaling questions. Select the questions that have the most relevance for you.

1. Would you consider yourself more religious or spiritual? Why?
2. How do your religious and spiritual beliefs and actions play out in your daily life? How does this relate to stress in your life?
3. Reflect on the times when you feel most spiritual. Where were you and what were you doing? What are you thinking and feeling?
4. What could you do today that would be a Random Act of Kindness (RAK)? And what could you do tomorrow ... and the next day ... and every day for the rest of your life? Discuss how your life, and the lives of those around you, would be changed if you incorporated RAKs into your daily life.
5. What do you currently do to grow in the spiritual dimension of health? If you were to implement a daily spiritual practice in your life, what would it be? How would you incorporate this practice into your daily life and why did you select this particular practice? How do you think this would decrease your stress and improve the quality of your life?
6. How does the information in this chapter affect you personally? What insights did you have about yourself and the stress that you experience?

ACTIVITY 2 - DVD EXERCISE - GUIDED IMAGERY - INNER WISDOM
(FOR MEDITATION AND INSIGHTS)

Objectives: The purpose of this activity is to allow you to experience personal insights gained through the guided imagery titled "Guided Imagery - Inner Wisdom."

Materials needed:
Stress Relief DVD, a quiet room, dim lighting
Handout 10:1 - Guided Imagery - Inner Wisdom
An extra CD player with some peaceful music - non-vocal new age or gentle classical music is best.

Description of Activity: Remain seated in your chair for this exercise.

Treat this exercise in a childlike manner - playfully and without expectations. If you aren't able to see the images as clearly as possible, simply sense the experience.

Insert the DVD into a DVD player and have in front of you Handout 10:1 - Guided Imagery - Inner Wisdom. Dim the lights or turn them off.

Start the DVD (cued to Guided Imagery - Inner Wisdom).

After this guided imagery has finished, turn on the lights and take a while to mindfully complete Handout 10:1.

Turn on some peaceful music as you write.

Handout 10:1 - Guided Imagery - Inner Wisdom
Following the guided imagery you just experienced, answer the two sets of questions below: (Note: If any part of the answer is too personal to write, then just say that it is too personal.) Use the other side of this page if you run out of room on this side.

What was your experience of meeting you as a child? Were you able to see yourself clearly? What thoughts were communicated between the two of you? What did you feel as you were with this child? How did it feel to leave?

What was the form of the being that you saw as your guide? Did you notice if it was a person or some other entity? If it was a person, did you recognize him or her? What was the communication that happened? What ideas, guidance, or insights did you receive from this guide?

ACTIVITY 3 - DVD RELAXATION EXERCISE - GUIDED IMAGERY - INNER WISDOM
(FOR RELAXATION)

Objectives: The purpose of this activity is to allow you to practice deep relaxation using the Guided Imagery - Inner Wisdom relaxation exercise

Materials needed:
Stress Relief DVD
DVD relaxation worksheet 10:2 titled DVD Relaxation Exercise - Guided Imagery - Inner Wisdom

Instructions:
1. Practice Guided Imagery - Inner Wisdom at least two times on your own.

2. Each time you finish, complete the instructional worksheet 10.2 called DVD Relaxation Exercise - Guided Imagery - Inner Wisdom.

3. If you do this experience in class, compare your experiences at home with your classroom experience.

4. This relaxation exercise is best done at times of the day other than right before going to sleep. The purpose of this particular relaxation exercise is not so much on helping you fall asleep as on helping you feel better, more relaxed, and refreshed.

DVD Relaxation Exercise
Handout 10:2 Guided Imagery - Inner Wisdom

The DVD homework assignment for this week is the fifth exercise on the Stress Relief DVD called "Guided Imagery - Inner Wisdom."

Practice doing this exercise at least two (2) times according to the instructions on the DVD. Resist the urge to fall asleep, so **don't** do it just before you go to bed.

Do it at times when you will not be disturbed. It lasts approximately 20 minutes.

In a *typed* format, respond to the following items:

1. How you felt before the exercise
2. Your experience during the exercise
3. How you felt immediately following the exercise
4. How you felt long after completing the exercise

On your typed paper, **thoroughly** respond to each of these items referring to the two times that you did them at home, *and* the time that you did it in class. Describe primarily how you were feeling in relation to your stress levels.

Follow this general outline with your description:

Daytime (first time):
- Before
- During
- Immediately after
- Long after

Daytime (second time):
- Before
- During
- Immediately after
- Long after

Classroom experience:
- Before
- During
- Immediately after
- Long after

ACTIVITY 4 - Spiritual Wellness Assessment

Objective: The purpose of this activity is to provide you with an opportunity to assess your spiritual wellness and to develop a personal plan to reduce stress through spiritual balance.

Instructions: Complete Handout 10:3 - Spiritual Wellness Assessment (also found in the text). The assessment has no right or wrong responses. It is intended to help you identify areas in which you may decide to do some spiritual growth work.

Handout 10:3 - Spiritual Wellness Assessment

Instructions: In front of each item below, choose one of the following:

S = I am *superior* in this area of my spiritual life

SS = I am doing *so-so* or okay in this area, but I could improve

NS = I *need strengthening* in this are (an area of growth for me)

_____ I have a deeply held belief system or personal theology.

_____ I have faith in a higher power.

_____ My faith gives meaning to the experiences and relations in my life.

_____ Even during difficult times, I have a sense of hope and peace.

_____ My spiritual beliefs help me remain calm and strong during times of stress.

_____ I feel a connection to the people and the world around me.

_____ I am able to forgive people, even when I think they have wronged me.

_____ I seek time with nature and reflect on how nature contributes to my quality of life.

_____ I find comfort in the practice of spiritual rituals (prayer, meditation, music).

_____ I feel loved.

_____ I am able to express my love for others freely.

_____ I respect the diversity of spiritual expression and am tolerant of those whose beliefs differ from my own.

_____ I can clearly articulate the meaning and purpose of my life.

_____ My inner strength is related to my belief in a higher power.

_____ I take time to be of service to others and enjoy doing so.

_____ I feel a sense of harmony and inner peace.

_____ I think my life is balanced.

_____ I feel responsible and am actively involved in preserving the environment.

_____ I see myself as a person of worth and feel comfortable with my own strengths and limitations.

_____ The way I live my life is a reflection of what I value most.

(Continued on next page.)

When you have completed the assessment questions, answer the following questions to help you with your spiritual growth:

1. What activities do you practice currently that help you feel spiritually healthy?

2. When all the surface layers of your life are peeled away, what do you believe makes up the core of your life — your purpose for being?

3. List two items from the Spiritual Wellness Assessment that you rated with an S and that you believe are most important for your spiritual well-being. Why are these items so important to you?

4. Of the items you rated *SS* or *NS*, which two do you think are most important for your spiritual growth?

5. What are three specific things you can do to grow spiritually for greater fulfillment and peace in your life?

Stress Less: Four Weeks to More Abundant Living, by M. Hesson (Nashville, TN: Abingdon Press, 1999).

ACTIVITY 5 - NEAR-DEATH EXPERIENCE

Objectives: The purpose of this activity is to give you the opportunity to investigate the amazing human phenomenon called the Near-Death Experience.

Materials needed:
Handout 10:4- Worksheet on the Near-Death Experience
Handout 10:5 - Near-Death Experience Questionnaire

Instructions:
Follow the instructions for completing this activity outlined below.

This activity deals with what is commonly known as the Near-Death Experience or NDE. This is a situation where someone has gone through what we would call death, but for whatever reason, he or she is resuscitated, or returns on their own, to normal life. While they are so-called "dead" their spirit seems to leave their body and pass through a number and variety of experiences. This exercise investigates those experiences.

Probably the best initial resources for information about the NDE can be found at these addresses:

http://www.iands.org/ This is the site of the International Association for Near-Death Studies.

and

http://www.near-death.com This site is packed with a huge assortment of interesting NDE's.

This activity has two parts.

1. Complete Handout 10:4- Worksheet on the Near-Death Experience. This will involve visiting the two websites and completely answering each of the questions. You may either write directly on the handout or create a typed version.

2. Next, complete Handout 10:5 - Near-Death Experience Questionnaire. Answering each of the questions, briefly relate a near-death experience that perhaps you or someone you know has had. This would be some experience that resembles those at the two websites.

If you do not personally know of anyone who has had a NDE, go to the websites, and find and read through some of the NDE's that are listed there. Briefly summarize one of their experiences. (DO NOT JUST COPY AND PASTE. Put it in your own words.)

Handout 10:4 Worksheet on the Near Death Experience

The first part of this assignment involves going to the following two websites:

www.near-death.com
www.iands.org

Based on the descriptions and case studies of Near Death Experiences (NDE), answer the following questions:

1. List ten of the common experiences that occur for people who have NDE's

2. Briefly describe ways that people's perspective on life, and their attitudes toward life, changes after they return from their NDE.

3. As you were reading, what came to mind as extremely interesting, unusual, or hard to believe?

Handout 10:5 Near Death Experience Questionnaire

This part of your assignment is to relate, briefly, a near-death experience that perhaps you or someone you know has had. This would be some experience that resembles those at the IANDS or the near-death.com websites.

If you do not know of anyone personally who has had an NDE, go to the IANDS or the near-death.com website, find and read some of the NDE's that are listed there. Briefly summarize one of their experiences.

Answer the following questions regarding the NDE:
1. How did they die? (What were the circumstances when they died or why did they die?)

2. What sequence of events happened to them once they noticed they were dead? Be specific and thorough.

3. What interesting feelings and thoughts did they report during their NDE?

4. What events or feelings that they report stand out to you as particularly fascinating?

5. What insights (if any) did they report about this earth life?

6. In what ways did they change (how were they different) when they returned from their NDE?

7. In what ways was their NDE the same and different from (compare and contrast) those you read on the websites?

RELATED WEBSITES

Spirituality and Health
HealthWorld Online's site for resources, links, and information on improving the our spiritual dimension
http://www.healthy.net/wellness/spirituality/

The New Trend in Health
Additional thoughts and spirituality as it relates to wellness
http://www.suite101.com/article.cfm/spirituality_health/115067

A study of university classroom strategies aimed at increasing spiritual health
The authors of this study proposed the research question: can spiritual health be enhanced through a planned educational intervention? Fascinating reading on spiritual health.
http://www.findarticles.com/p/articles/mi_m0FCR/is_4_37/ai_112720424

CHAPTER 11
TIME AND LIFE MANAGEMENT

CHAPTER OUTLINE
Use this outline to take notes as you read the chapter in the text and/or as your instructor lectures in class.

I.   **TIME AND LIFE MANAGEMENT**
  A. Time management is about taking action.
      1. The perception that we don't have enough time is one of life's great stressors.
      2. We all have exactly 60 minutes in every hour, 24 hours in every day, and 168 hours in every week.
      3. Time management is really about managing our self and our life to do and have the things that are most important to us.

II. **WHAT IS TIME MANAGEMENT?**
  A. Time is the medium through which our lives are lived.
      1. How we choose to spend our time determines the level of satisfaction we experience.
  B. **Time** is the occurrence of all of the events of our lives, one after another.
  C. **Management** is the art or manner of controlling.
  D. **Time management**, therefore, is the art or manner of controlling the sequence of events in our lives.

III. **TIME AND STRESS**
  A. Time is one of those areas of life where we often feel like we have lost control.
  B. Gaining some control over how we use our time is crucial to managing stress.
      1. Both low and high time pressure can have a negative impact on mental health.
      2. People with a perceived sense of control over their time and their life experience less stress.
  C. Men and women spend time differently (see Graph 11-1).
      1. Women are twice as likely as men to indicate they feel frequently overwhelmed by all they have to do.

IV. **PLANNING FOR CONTROL**
  A. The way that we gain control of our lives is by planning.
      1. **Planning** is the act of bringing future events into the present so appropriate control can be applied.
  B. **Pareto's Law** says that, in many activities, 80% of the potential value can be achieved from just 20% of the effort, and that one can spend the remaining 80% of effort for relatively little return.
      1. The reverse is also true- things that take up 80% of your time and resources will only produce 20% of your results.
      2. Concentrating your efforts on the key activities that get results will increase your efficiency and decrease your stress.
          a) You have the power to set the vital priorities which will mean the difference between failure, survival, and success.
  C. Methods of time management
      1. Most methods of planning and time management begin by asking these four crucial questions:
          a) What are my highest priorities? (What is most important to me?)
          b) Of my priorities, which do I value the most?
          c) What can I do about my highest priorities in the days and weeks to come?
          d) When, during today or this week, will I do these things?

2. No time management system works equally well for everyone.
   a) Each of the time management methods in this chapter has been found to be effective in helping people gain control over their lives and significantly reduce their stress as a result.

V. ABC123 PRIORITIZED PLANNING
   A. The focus of this method is to move from crisis management and putting out fires toward doing those things that are most important to us on a daily basis.
      1. The first part of this process is deciding to dedicate 15 minutes each day to the process of thoughtful planning according to three phases or steps.
   B. Phase I - Make a List.
      1. Write down everything you want to accomplish today.
      2. This looks much like a traditional to-do list.
   C. Phase II - Give a value to each item on the list using ABC.
      1. Put an "A" next to each item on your list that *must* be done today.
         a) These are the vital things that have the highest amount of importance to you.
      2. Place a "B" by each item that should be done today.
         a) These are items with *some importance* to you.
      3. Place a "C" by each item that has *very little importance* to you.
         a) These items could be done, but won't suffer at all if they are not.
      4. The value you give items will change with the events in your life.
         a) The key point is that you are the one who is evaluating the relative importance of each of the items on your list based on how you currently perceive them.
   D. Phase III - Prioritize again using 123
      1. Give a numerical value to each item on the list based on its relative importance to you.
         a) Move through the "A" items and compare each one.
         b) Ask yourself which of these very important items is *the most important of all*.
         c) That item gets a "1" next to the "A" so it becomes "A1" on your list.
         d) Proceed through each of the A's until you have given a ranking to each.
         e) Then proceed to the B's and then the C's.
   E. There is a very real human tendency to skip the most valuable and important things (the "A" items on the list) and move to those items that are easier, more fun, or less demanding (the "B" and "C" items on the list).
      1. There are consequences for choosing to do this.
         a) Many of your important items will turn into urgent items.
            (1) This is the urgency mode called "putting out the fires."
         b) The other consequence is inner chaos.
            (1) When we do the things that are most important to us, we experience inner peace because what we do and what we value are aligned.
            (2) When we don't do those things that are aligned with what we value, we lose our inner peace.
   F. On most days, you won't finish everything on your list. In fact, you rarely do.
      1. The real value of this system becomes clear when we have periods of free time where we can choose between several activities.
         a) It is in those parts of the day that we can go to the top of our list, our A1 item, and work from there.

VI. QUADRANT PLANNING
   A. First Things First
      1. Quadrant planning begins with a more long-term approach to time management by

inviting you to first answer some questions.
- a) Are the things that are less important in your life receiving the most attention?
- b) Are too many good things getting in the way of your best?
- c) Are you making the tough decision to choose the best over the good?
- d) What activities, if you know you did superbly and consistently, would have a significant positive impact on your life?
- e) How many people, on their deathbed, wish they had spent more time at the office?

2. We should first ask ourselves, "Am I doing the right things?"
   - a) After we have answered this question, we can ask, "Am I doing things right?"

B. Urgency Versus Importance
1. The key to doing first things first is to distinguish between the urgent and the important.
   - a) We may be busy working as hard as we can only to find that at the end of the day, we feel unfulfilled.
     - (1) This is because we put the **urgent** - those things demanding our attention in the moment - before the **important** – the things that would make a difference long-term.
   - b) The only way to truly master our time is to organize our schedules each day such that we spend the majority of our time doing things that are important but not necessarily urgent.
2. Quadrant 2 activities are the important activities and should be our first things; the things on which we focus most of our time and energy. (See Figure 11-2 Activity Matrix).
   - a) The metaphor of the rocks suggests that if we don't put in the big rocks first - the most important things - they won't make it into the jar and don't get considered.

C. Quadrant Planning in Action
1. Step I – Quadrant 2 Questions
   - a) Several questions invite us to first ask ourselves about the more important things:
     - (1) What do I want to be, do, and contribute in my life?
     - (2) What three or four things are most important to me?
     - (3) What are my long-range goals?
     - (4) Which relationships are most important to me?
     - (5) What are my main responsibilities?
     - (6) What contributions would I like to make?
     - (7) What are the principles that I value?
     - (8) What feelings do I want to experience in life?
     - (9) How would I spend the coming week if I only had 6 months to live?

       (a) The answers to these questions should guide us in deciding our daily activities.

2. Step 2: Identify Roles
   - a) Much pain comes from the realization that we are succeeding in one role at the expense of another.
     - (1) Too often we hear of people who are very successful in their business life but they encounter problems with their family life or their spiritual life.
   - b) A holistic view of life involves a balance between the various dimensions of life including the physical, social, mental, emotional, and spiritual.
   - c) Our roles help us fulfill the needs of these dimensions and give us a sense

of wholeness of a quality of life.
    d) These roles may include family, personal, business, school, relationships, and community.
        (1) Ask the question: What is the most important thing I can do in this role today or this week to have the greatest positive impact in my life?
  3. Step 4: Sharpen the Saw
    a) Taking time to sharpen your saw (life enhancing activities) can dramatically affect the level of accomplishment you feel in your life.
    b) There are things in life we can do that, if we did them on a regular basis, would help us to sharpen our saw and allow us to do all the other things that we do with greater ease and effectiveness.
        (1) Exercising, eating well, managing stress, getting sufficient sleep, studying good literature, practicing forgiveness, attending religious services are all examples.
  4. Step 4: Evaluate - How Did I Do?
    a) **Integrity** is the ability to carry out a worthy decision after the emotion of making the decision has passed.
        (1) It is very easy, when we are in the silence of our planning sessions, to design our days and weeks according to our conscience and according to the things that we feel are most important.
        (2) The challenge is to keep the first things first in this moment of choice.
            (b) As we are proceeding through our day according to our plan, someone encourages us to do something that is of far less importance, though it may seem very enticing.
            (c) Are we going to sacrifice the best for the good in that moment?
    b) At the end of the day, part of our movement toward developing ourselves, reducing stress, and reaching our goals involves assessing what we have done to help us move toward each of these with integrity.
    c) Evaluation is the art of looking back and seeing what we did, how we did it, and if it worked to produce the results that we intended.

VII. **LIFEBALANCE: A MORE FLOWING APPROACH TO TIME AND LIFE MANAGEMENT**
  A. Critics of traditional time management approaches contend that more rigid planning tends to focus too much on doing and having, and not enough on being.
    1. If we have planned every minute of our day and if we do not cross off every planned action from our list, we feel like we have failed.
    2. These approaches do not appear to allow for spontaneity, freedom, and "going with the flow."
      a) To some, there is emptiness to the traditional approaches.
  B. **Lifebalance** is an approach to time and life management that promotes a balance of purposeful planning and a healthy mix of going with the flow.
  C. Unbalance, according to Richard and Linda Eyre, results from bad habits - habits that emphasize work at the expense of family and personal growth, structure at the expense of spontaneity, or accomplishments at the expense of relationships (or vice versa on any of these).
    1. The result of this imbalance is what Thoreau called "lives of quiet desperation."
  D. The search for simpler, slower, more flexible and more meaningful lives has vanished in our culture with the constant search for *more*, *better*, and *different*.
    1. Contentedness has been replaced by competition.
    2. Serenity has been replaced by speed.
  E. Balance implies a healthy combination of all that is important to us and letting our inner

nature, rather than our environment and culture, dictate our speed and direction.
   F. The current frustration and dilemma that many feel with time management planners include:
      1. Ninety-five percent of what is written in planners has to do with work, career, or finance creating an imbalance between work and family and personal needs.
      2. Planners cause us to live by lists, to act rather than respond. If we're not careful, our lists control us rather than the other way around. We begin to view things that are not on our lists as irrelevant, or distractions rather than as opportunities, and we begin to lose the critical balance between structure and spontaneity.
      3. Because they are accomplishment-oriented, most planners focus their attention on things, on getting, and on doing, sometimes at the expense of people and giving and thinking, resulting in an imbalance between achievements and relationships.

VIII. KEYS TO CREATING BALANCE
   A. Simplifying
      1. When we sit down to plan, rather than asking, "What do I have to do?" we ask different questions, such as, "What do I *choose* to do? Or "What do I *want* to do?"
      2. The ability to simplify our days, and our lives, can be developed by regularly asking these four questions:
         a) Will it matter in 10 years?
         b) What do I need more of in my life?
         c) What do I need less of?
         d) How can I make this simpler?
      3. Continually adding more things to our life frequently complicates and speeds up the pace of our life.
      4. Removing things from our lives creates simplicity and freedom.
   B. Doing What Really Matters
      1. Focus our priorities on three specific areas, then work to balance these areas.
         a) Family: This area includes our relationships with family and friends.
         b) Work/Career/School: This area includes all areas of our professional development.
         c) Self: This area includes not only development with our inner self, but the way we function serving others, including activity with church and community groups.
   C. Don't Just Do Something—Sit there!
      1. Planning our days involves a commitment to stop everything and spend at least 5 minutes stopping and doing nothing other than thinking.
      2. Rather than asking, "What do I really want?" Ask challenging but perhaps more useful questions such as: What do I need?" "What do I need in my physical, social, spiritual, intellectual, and emotional life?"
         a) Choose the thing you need to do most and do it that day..
   D. Balancing Attitude--Balance structure with spontaneity.
      1. Attitude balance involves considering both the destination and the journey.
         a) Our culture thrives on reaching goals and enjoying the good feeling that comes with accomplishment.
         b) We tend to frequently forget about the joy of the journey and the footsteps we take on the way to the goal, which are just as important as the goal itself.
      2. **Antiplanning** describes the attitude of making goals, being firm about where we want to go, but at the same time, being flexible on how we are to get there.
         a) We don't always know, with our limited wisdom, what is the best way to do something.
            (1) If we remain open to opportunities, rather than staying rigidly attached to what we have planned, we may find new directions, new opportunities, and sometimes even better goals that present

themselves.

    b) Antiplanning shifts our focus to a simpler attitude of enjoying each step of the journey as much as the goal that we will reach.

    3. Freeing the mind, when we come up with our best ideas, happens in those times when our thinking has slowed and we aren't focusing on anything in particular.

        a) Examples of these times include when we are in the shower, daydreaming, sleeping in, taking a leisurely solo stroll, or driving.

        b) Often these insights can completely change an entire day or an entire lifetime toward a more fulfilling and joyful experience.

            (1) If we don't let the ideas through because of the busy-ness of our minds, we miss out on these best things.

IX. SERENDIPITY

    A. Closely related to the Lifebalance approach to time management is the idea of **serendipity** that describes the quality which, through good fortune and sagacity, allows a person to discover something good while seeking something else.

    B. The Three Princes of Serendipity

        1. The essence of this principle learned by the three Princes of Serendip is that the happenings you never expect are actually the things that are supposed to happen. Other definitions for serendipity include:

            a) The capacity for making happy and unexpected discoveries by accident.

            b) The gift of finding valuable or agreeable things not sought for.

            c) An unexpected discovery of something worthwhile during a search of an expected something worthwhile.

    C. The Keys to serendipity

        1. The first is that we need to be working toward something.

            a) We need to set some goal(s) for ourselves and be moving in the direction of them.

        2. The second feature of serendipity is that we need to be aware, to be alert, to be observing things in order to realize the so-called "happy accidents" that occur as we are on the way to our original goal.

            a) If we aren't tuning in to what is happening, we will miss things like beauty, spontaneous moments, new and even better goals and directions, opportunities, and needs of others as they arise.

    D. Applying Serendipity

        1. Knowing about serendipity and applying the principle in daily life are two very different things.

        2. Serendipity is not a common way of being for most people in our culture.

    E. Split-page Scheduling

        1. Start your planning time by drawing a line down the middle of your daily planning page.

            a) The left side of this page is our traditional scheduling of activities and planning items to do that day.

            b) The right side of the page is left blank.

                (1) This side will be filled, during the day or at the end of the day, with those unanticipated needs, unforeseen opportunities, and the unexpected moments that come up during the day.

                (2) These are the items that we could not have planned for, but turn out to be as valuable, or more valuable, than the things that we had planned.

            c) The left side gets the list; the right side gets the day's serendipitous after-it-happens notes, such as a new acquaintance, a fresh idea, a child's question, an unexpected opportunity, a friend's need, a chance meeting, a beautiful sunset.

            d) We have to be in pursuit of something (left side of the page) and we have to be aware, sensitive, and observant of those other things that we didn't plan for (right side of the page).

   e) The right side of the page reminds us to be playful, spontaneous, risk-taking, and serendipitous.

F. The guiding principle of Lifebalance and Serendipity is to be *"strong and fixed on the destination, but be creative and flexible on the route."* (See Box 11-1 Gaining the Quality of Serendipity)

X. PROCRASTINATION

A. **Procrastination** is the avoidance of a task which needs to be accomplished.
   1. This can lead to feelings of guilt, inadequacy, depression, and self-doubt. Procrastination has a high potential for painful consequences.
   2. It interferes with our academic, professional, and personal success.

B. Linda Sapadin identifies six styles of procrastination.
   1. Perfectionists fear that they can't complete tasks up to their expectations.
      a) They focus on details rather than overall objectives, and they fear making mistakes.
   2. Dreamers have big goals but fail to translate their ideas into a plan for action.
      a) They contrast with perfectionists because dreamers never get to the details.
   3. Worriers focus on the worst case scenario and see the problems rather than the solutions.
      a) They tend to avoid change and risk-taking.
   4. Crisis makers wait until the pressure mounts to take action.
      a) By waiting until the last minute to complete a task, they create excitement from a temporary rush of adrenaline – and put their projects at risk.
   5. Defiers resist new tasks and often don't follow through on what they promise to do.
      a) They avoid team work and are reluctant to make agreements.
   6. Overdoers make the job harder than it needs to be and create extra work.
      a) They fail to set priorities and refuse to delegate.

C. Tips for overcoming the procrastination habit:
   1. Turn elephants into hors d'oeuvres:
      a) Cut a huge task into smaller chunks so it seems less enormous.
   2. Avoid Cramming
      a) The single most important key to improving grades may be **distributed study** time: spacing your learning periods with rest periods between sessions. Cramming is called **massed study**. Studies indicate that distributed study is superior to massed study for memory and learning.
   3. Manage your time zappers:
      a) A significant deterrent to successful time management is **time zappers**, those things that take time away from what is more important.
         (1) Probably the most significant time zapper is television viewing.
   4. Work hardest during your "best times" of the day
      a) Most of us have two or three hours during the day when we are the most productive.
         (1) Try to schedule your time so that your most important activities can be done during these "best times" of the day.
   5. Keep an activity log
      a) You may be surprised at how much time you spend doing things that might be considered a waste of time or have little value for you or anyone else.
   6. Choose to refuse
      a) Say "NO" to the unimportant or less important things.
      b) Saying "no" to extra projects, social activities, and invitations you know you don't have the time or energy for can prevent a lot of unnecessary worry, guilt, and wasted emotional energy down the road.

7. Try delegating
   a) If some things do not require your personal attention, delegate them to someone else.
8. Establish levels of acceptable perfection
   a) Take a realistic look at your tasks and determine which can be your "good" work and which should be your "best."
      (1) Frequently, there are things we do that don't necessarily require high degrees of perfection.
      (2) When this is the case, complete the task at an appropriate level depending upon the importance of the item.
9. Do the most difficult or most unpleasant tasks first
   a) Once you have the tough tasks out of the way, you are freer to enjoy your other tasks that are more pleasant and fun.
10. Use "wasted" time
    a) Time we spend sitting in the doctor's office or waiting for an oil change can be useful downtime.
11. Enjoy the process
    a) Ask yourself how you can do the task *AND* have fun in the process.
    b) If you know that something has to be done, but is unpleasant to even think about, ask yourself how you can add something enjoyable to the process.
12. Reward yourself
    a) Promise yourself a reward for completing each task, or finishing the entire task.
    b) Then keep your promise to yourself and indulge in your reward.
       (1) Doing so will help you maintain the necessary balance between work and play.
13. Let some things go undone
    a) Let it be okay to not finish some things, and even to not do some things that are on your list.
    b) You decide what can be left undone and you can allow yourself to be okay with that.

XI. CONCLUSION

A. In the final analysis, how you spend your time, and what events you participate in every moment of each day, is your choice.
B. As you make those choices, don't mistake activity for achievement.
   1. Take time to pause from time to time and remind yourself of where you are going and how you want to get there.
C. The time management systems in this chapter are designed to help you gain more control of your life and thereby reduce your stress and enhance your well-being.
   1. You will find that planning sets you free.
D. In the end, time management is really more about managing yourself and your life than it is about managing time.
   1. "I don't have enough time" is replaced by "I have plenty of time for what matters to me."

<u>LEARNING ACTIVITIES</u>

ACTIVITY 1 - JOURNALING

Objective: The purpose of this activity is to encourage critical thinking and honest personal reflection on topics relating to the chapter content. Explore personal thoughts, feelings, values, and behaviors as you selectively incorporate stress management knowledge and behaviors into your plan for improved health through better stress management.

Instructions: You will find journaling questions in each chapter of your Activities Manual. These questions relate specifically to the chapter content. Moving your thoughts from your mind to the paper is a powerful strategy for relieving stress and for increasing awareness of your thoughts, feelings and behaviors. Your course instructor can provide further guidance on how to complete this activity.

Complete the following journaling questions. Select the questions that have the most relevance for you.

1. What does it mean to you to manage your time?
2. What do you think are the main differences between "doing things right" and "doing the right thing." Think of an example that might illustrate how you may be doing things right and yet not be doing the right things.
3. What would you say are your greatest time zappers? How can you swap time zappers for time spent on something more important to you?
4. Of the three methods of managing time described in this chapter, which is the most appealing to you? Why?
5. What things can you do specifically to Sharpen Your Saw?
6. Think about the major roles in your life. Which ones seem to need more attention so that your life feels more fulfilling?
7. Look through the list on Overcoming Procrastination - Tips on Time Management. Pick out two things from the list that most relate to you. How can you include these tips in your daily activities?
8. Think of a time when you experienced serendipity, that is, something happened seemingly by chance, but turned out to be a better path than you were planning to take. How did you feel when this happened?
9. How does the information in this chapter affect you personally? What insights did you have about yourself and the stress that you experience?

ACTIVITY 2 - TIME LOG

Objectives: The purpose of this activity is to give you the experience of seeing exactly how you spend your time.

Materials needed:
Handout 11:1 - Activity/Time Log

Description of Activity: For 3 or 4 consecutive days, keep track of every waking moment. Follow the Activity/Time Log as a guide to see how it is to be done. Be sure to include each activity or every minute of your day.

Once you have completed this for 3 or 4 days, analyze how you can use your time more effectively.

Handout 11:1 - Activity/Time Log

Date	Time of Day	Time Spent	Purpose/Activity

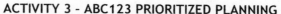

ACTIVITY 3 - ABC123 PRIORITIZED PLANNING

Objectives: The purpose of this activity is to allow you to practice time management and planning according to the ABC123 Prioritized Daily Planning Method.

Materials needed:
Handout 11:2 - Prioritized Daily Planning
Blank pieces of paper

Description of Activity: Consider today as you work on this exercise. Move through each of the phases on the handout writing down all of your information on the blank piece of paper.

Refer to the information in chapter 11 for further details about this process.

ACTIVITY 4 - ABC123 PRIORITIZED PLANNING - EXTENDED PRACTICE

Objectives: The purpose of this activity is to give you extended daily practice using the ABC123 Prioritized Daily Planning Method.

Materials needed:
Handout 11:2 - Prioritized Daily Planning
Handout 11:3 - ABC123 Prioritized Daily Planning Method Assessment
Paper, notebook, or a planner available at most bookstores

Description of Activity: For the next 3 weeks, plan each day according to the ABC123 Prioritized Planning method. You can do this in the evening prior to the following day or in the morning before the events of the day. At the end of 3 weeks, complete Handout 11:3.

Refer to the information in chapter 11 for further details about this process.

Handout 11:2 - Prioritized Daily Planning

Planning is bringing future events into the present so appropriate control can be applied.The most valuable thing we can do to positively impact our days is spend 10-15 minutes planning. Ultimately, we always do exactly what we want to do.

We are answering and acting on these key questions:
- What are my highest priorities? What do I value most?
- What can I do about these most important things today and this week?

Phases of Planning:
Phase I - Cross out non-discretionary time
Consider all those times during the day when you have agreed with yourself or someone else that you will participate in a particular activity to the exclusion of all other things.
- Meetings, classes, work, study groups, dinnertime with family, sporting events, exercise time, etc.

Phase II - Consider our Roles
We all have several roles
- Individual, spouse, employee, student, athlete, family member, community/church member, friend, etc.

Phase III - Ask: What are the most important things I can do in relation to each of these roles?
We begin answering the questions above with this question: What can we do in each of our roles that would significantly add value to the role? How can we improve in each role?
- Some days we will think of several things that we can do for our roles.
- Some days we may not be able to think of anything for a particular role.
- We must think of those most important things FIRST before considering our other activities of the day.

Phase IV - Make a list of daily tasks. Include those from Phase III
This begins to look like a To-Do list.
Unload your mind of everything that comes to mind to be done today.
Include all of those things that came to mind in Phase III.

Phase V - Give a letter to each item on your list
A - Must be done - these are highly important/vital.
- These aren't the urgent things. Urgency is reactive mode.

B - Should be done - these are fairly important
C - Could be done - these hare not vital, and not very important

Phase VI - Give a numerical value to each item on the list.
Begin with A items
- Highest priority gets a 1, next gets a 2, next gets a 3, and so on.

We are determining the order, the sequence of what we will do during the day, based on what we have determined are the most important things in our lives.

Phase VII - Exercise Integrity
Character is the ability to carry out a worthy decision after the emotion of making the decision has passed.

Handout 11:3 – ABC123 Prioritized Daily Planning Method Assessment
Name _____

Please answer each question as honestly and accurately as possible:

1. On a scale from 0 to 10, rate how frequently and correctly (according to the instructions you were given to plan each day) you followed the directions for your prioritized daily planning. (0 = you didn't try even once to follow the directions to plan and follow through since it was introduced to you. 10 = you planned every day and followed through with your plan as perfectly as possible) Place your score on the following line:

_____

2. How much of a difference did this activity make for you? Did you have more control over your time? Did you experience more inner peace? Did you accomplish more? What else did you notice about this? Do you plan to continue using this method of time management or some variation of it? Why or why not?

RELATED WEBSITES

Managing Your Time
This site provides you with tips for managing your time well so you can get the most out of your college experience.
http://www.dartmouth.edu/~acskills/success/time.html

Where Does Time Go?
Complete this short questionnaire to see how much time you really have available to study for your classes.
http://www.ucc.vt.edu/stdysk/TMInteractive.html

Ten Tips You Need to Survive College
Your first-aid kit--10 tips to keep you afloat
http://www.mtsu.edu/%7Estudskl/10tips.html

CHAPTER 12
MONEY MATTERS

CHAPTER OUTLINE
Use this outline to take notes as you read the chapter in the text and/or as your instructor lectures in class.

I. **MONEY MATTERS**
   A. This chapter relates to one of the most common stressors around the world - not enough money.
      1. While it is true that money won't make you happy, lack of money is one of life's great stressors.
      2. In this chapter you will complete a series of exercises to start you on the road to financial fitness.
      3. You will learn how to manage your money so you can reduce your stress now and for years to come.
   B. Financial pressure ranks high in the list of stressors facing college students.
      1. Financial problems rank right up there with poor grades as the major reasons for dropping out of college.
      2. There are some specific exercises that can help you develop financial fitness.

II. **ABCS OF MONEY MANAGEMENT**
   A. Assessment - Assessment means looking at where you are right now and evaluating how you got there.
      1. Begin by becoming more aware of both your current spending habits and the thoughts and emotions linked to spending.
      2. To get started, keep track of what you spend for one week.
         a) For now, don't worry about your monthly expenses; just record your daily spending for a full week, including a weekend.
      3. Thoughts and emotions linked to money - Assessment includes not just tracking where our money goes, but also assessing why we spend money.
         a) Have you ever gone out and bought something expensive when you were sad or lonely as a way to try to feel better?
         b) Begin to notice how often issues of stress and money are related.
   B. A **budget** is a plan you develop to manage your money so you can have what is most important to you and accomplish your financial goals.
      1. First write your financial goals and then develop a plan to accomplish those goals. Writing **SMART goals** will increase the likelihood of accomplishing your goals.
         a) Write your financial goals with a focus on your college years.
         b) Include both short-term and long-term goals for your years as a student.
      2. Once you have written your financial goals, look back to Exercise 1 where you recorded everything you spent for a week.
         a) Take a red pen and cross out all the expenditures that were unnecessary and that did not contribute to your financial goals.
      3. Calculate what you expect your income to be over the academic year.
         a) Add up all sources of money, including from your work, financial aid, and from your family.
      4. Next, determine your expenses for the year.
      5. Develop your budget by following these steps:
         a) Get your checkbook, credit card statements, or other records of expenditures.
         b) Make columns for each category of spending; for example, tuition, food, rent, entertainment, and car expenses.
         c) List, as best you can, each purchase under the proper column. Use dollar amounts only.

d) Total each column.
e) Add every column total together.
f) Compare this with your income.
g) Make adjustments where necessary.

C. Control - Now that you can clearly see the money coming in and the money going out, you can begin to make informed choices on how to balance your financial situation to accomplish your financial goals and, as a result, experience less stress and greater satisfaction.

1. A budget suggests that you have some fixed expenses, like tuition or car payments, and you have some flexible expenses, like going out to eat or buying a new shirt.
   a) Differentiate between what you want and what you truly need.
   b) Even though it doesn't always feel like it, you have choices about both income and expenditures.
2. Your budget is not just recording income and expenses, but consciously deciding how you will manage your money.

III. **DOODADS AND CREDIT CARDS**

A. **Doodads** are small but steady expenses that can drain away our cash. This is sometimes called the **latte factor**.

1. We waste a lot of money by not thinking carefully about the purchases we make.
2. Eliminating doodads can go a long way in improving your peace of mind.
3. The intention is not to eliminate the special things that bring pleasure to life, but to thoughtfully analyze where you are spending your money to determine if the costs are worth the benefits.

B. Credit cards can be an especially subtle way to accumulate debt.

1. Financial advisors estimate that we would spend about 20 percent less just by switching to a cash-only payment system.
2. Here are tips for managing credit:
   a) Use credit cards only for emergencies or carefully planned-in-advance purchases.
   b) If you must use a credit card, make every effort to pay off the full balance each month.
   c) Limit yourself to one credit card. Do you really need the free t-shirt or clock radio that credit card companies are giving away to get you to sign up?
   d) Remember that credit is DEBT and not supplementary income.
   e) Do not pay just the minimum payment each month. Paying even $20 or $25 more than the minimum can save you thousands of dollars over time.
   f) Try to get a credit card with a lower interest rate (see author's anecdote).
   g) Learning to defer gratification is an important aspect of money management. Avoid impulse buying by making your money or credit card hard to obtain. Leave your credit card home or take only a pre-determined amount of money with you when you go out.
   h) Try wrapping your credit card and securing it with tape when you carry it with you. Just the act of unwrapping it might allow you time to reconsider if you really need to make this purchase.
   i) Limit the amount you can put on your card every month - it's a budget, simply put.
   j) Be aware that student credit card deals aren't always your best bet. As a student with a limited credit history you're considered a credit risk, so although you may get the card, you'll probably have a high interest rate.
   k) Rather than a credit card, use only a debit card where the money is coming right out of your checking account. That way, you can't spend more than you have.

3. Credit cards can also serve a valuable function if used carefully. Weigh the pros and cons carefully.
    a) Pros
        (1) Establish a good credit rating so if in the future I need to buy something big, like a home or car, I will be able to secure a loan.
        (2) A credit card could save the day if a true emergency arises and I need money fast.
        (3) Some credit cards include insurance for the items I purchase.
        (4) A credit card might come in handy so I don't always have to carry cash.
    b) Cons
        (1) I might spend more money with a credit card because it doesn't seem like real money.
        (2) Interest rates can be very high so if I can't pay off the balance. I might end up throwing my money away on interest.
        (3) The fine print on the credit card agreement can be impossible to understand. I may not know what I am getting into.
        (4) If I can't keep up on my payments, I can mess up my credit rating for 7 years (or more).

IV. ADDITIONAL TIPS FOR MANAGING YOUR MONEY
   A. See chapter 12 for a list of additional ideas given by students to prevent or reduce financial stress.

V. CAN MONEY MAKE YOU HAPPY?
   A. The source of much stress is not just money itself, but rather the value we give to money.
       1. Stress-relieving money management may be just as much about managing our mind as about managing our money.
   B. Even though we have more income per capita, more things, bigger houses and more toys than we had 50 years ago, about one third of Americans describe themselves as "very happy" and the percentage remains almost exactly the same today as it was in the 1950s.
       1. Many people mistakenly believe that more money means greater happiness.
       2. There is not a significant relationship between how much money a person earns and whether he or she feels good about life.
   C. We live in a culture that encourages consumerism and overspending.
       1. This ongoing battle with consumerism can lead to a dangerous trap - living beyond our means.
       2. The more we make, the more we spend. This epidemic to want more and spend money we don't have is called **affluenza**.
   D. Some of the financial distress we experience is really of our own making.
       1. Sociologists describe **reference anxiety** as what happens when people judge their possessions in comparison with others, not based on what they need.
           a) When we gauge our happiness on that comparison, we end up chasing money rather than meaning.
           b) The outcome is stress, frustration and dissatisfaction with what we have.
           c) Money no longer provides a sense of well-being, even when we have more than an adequate amount to meet our needs.
   E. Money is a source of stress in many relationships.
       1. It is not just the perceived shortage of money, but also the time we spend making money rather than being with family and friends, as well as disagreements on how money should be used.
       2. Once our basic needs are met, it is not necessarily the money, or lack of it, that causes us stress.
           a) It is how we think about money that determines the role it plays in our well-being.
           b) We determine the value we give to money and as a result, either the

satisfaction or distress it produces.

    3. After a certain level of income is reached, happiness and money don't seem to have much relationship to each other.

        a) Placing too much value on money can be a source of unnecessary fear and distress.

VI. CONCLUSION

    A. Changing how you spend and save money can be challenging, but can bring a lifetime of financial freedom.

    B. There is more to money that just earning and spending.

        1. Money is often connected with feelings and wealth is mistakenly believed to be the road to happiness.

        2. Not having adequate money can and does contribute to stress, but remember that money in and of itself is no assurance of happiness.

        3. Money is neither good nor bad; it is simply a tool, just as a pencil is a tool.

            a) While a pencil is designed to write with, it can also be used as a lethal weapon to stab a person in the eye.

            b) The thing that makes the difference isn't the object, but the motives of the person holding the pencil - or handling the money.

LEARNING ACTIVITIES

ACTIVITY 1 - JOURNALING

Objective: The purpose of this activity is to encourage critical thinking and honest personal reflection on topics relating to the chapter content. Explore personal thoughts, feelings, values, and behaviors as you selectively incorporate stress management knowledge and behaviors into your plan for improved health through better stress management.

Instructions: You will find journaling questions in each chapter of your Activities Manual. These questions relate specifically to the chapter content. Moving your thoughts from your mind to the paper is a powerful strategy for relieving stress and for increasing awareness of your thoughts, feelings and behaviors. Your course instructor can provide further guidance on how to complete this activity.

Complete the following journaling questions. Select the questions that have the most relevance for you.

1. Reflect on money management strategies that have helped you reduce your financial distress. Ask your parents or other adults based on their experience what advice they would offer. List your top tips for money management. Rank your list and think about why you rank them in this order.
2. How do you think money can be used to try to deal with emotions like loneliness or as a way to feel more powerful? Can you identify times when you used money to deal with your emotional needs? Assess the emotions that you were dealing with (power, loneliness, anger, love). What are problems that come to mind associated with using money to cope with emotional issues? What are ways other than spending money for dealing with these emotions?
3. What are some effective ways you can reduce stress and have fun without spending money?
4. Discuss the exercises you did for this chapter. Which ones were most helpful to you? What did you learn?
5. How does the information in this chapter affect you personally? What insights did you have about yourself and the stress that you experience?

ACTIVITY 2 - SPENDING HABITS AND EMOTIONS

Objective: The purpose of this activity is to provide you with an opportunity to track your spending habits and to increase awareness of emotions that influence spending.

Instructions: Complete Handout 12:1 - Spending Habits and Emotions.

HANDOUT 12:1 - SPENDING HABITS AND EMOTIONS

Name: _____

Directions: For one week, keep track of everything you spend. At the end of the week, go back and review your log and answer the questions at the end of the handout. Make additional copies of the log as needed. Note whether the purchase is a "want" or a "need." Ask yourself this question, "Is this purchase something I truly need or is it something I would just like to have?" Also, assess your emotions at the time of purchase. Were you happy, depressed, lonely, or bored? Try not to change your spending habits during the week you complete the log. Let this serve as a record of your normal spending habits.

DATE, DAY, TIME	PLACE	AMOUNT SPENT	WHAT YOU PURCHASED	WANT OR NEED	EMOTIONS ASSOCIATED WITH PURCHASE

Reflection Questions: After you have completed your spending log for one week, review your log and answer these questions:

1. Do you notice any patterns to your spending behaviors? For example, do you spend more money when you are with certain people or at certain times of the day?

2. What do you notice about your emotions related to spending?

3. Are there any purchases that you made this week that you now regret making?

4. Do your spending habits contribute to your stress? If so, how and what changes can you make to help you reduce financial stress?

5. List 3 things you learned from completing this assignment.

ACTIVITY 3 - FINANCIAL GOALS

Objective: The purpose of this activity is to provide you with an opportunity to write your financial goals.

Instructions: Review the SMART format for writing goals. Write both short term financial goals for this school year and longer term goals for when you finish college. Think about how having financial goals can help reduce stress.

<u>**RELATED WEBSITES**</u>

Young Money - Money Management
Great website devoted to all things financial for the college student.
http://www.youngmoney.com/

Financial Fitness Tools
A website aimed at educating college students about personal finance. You can determine if you are financially fit, get advice on the wise use of credit cards, learn how to avoid defaulting on your student loan and other debts, and access information on credit reports and investment options. It also provides interactive calculators to help you with budgeting, balancing a checkbook, savings, and loan consolidation.
http://www.mapping-your-future.org/features/dmtensteps.htm

7 steps for building financial fitness
Would you be able to financially survive a job loss or a medical emergency? When life deals those unexpected hurdles, you want to be as prepared as possible. Check out these strategies for curbing debts and building savings.
http://www.bankrate.com/brm/news/special/20020726a.asp

CHAPTER 13
SOCIAL SUPPORT, RELATIONSHIPS, AND COMMUNICATION

CHAPTER OUTLINE
Use this outline to take notes as you read the chapter in the text and/or as your instructor lectures in class.

I. **SOCIAL SUPPORT, RELATIONSHIPS, AND COMMUNICATION**
    A. Friends are good medicine, especially when it comes to preventing stress.
        1. It is well known that social support and close relationships go hand-in-hand with good health.
            a) Studies indicate that loneliness has the opposite effect.
        2. Supportive relationships can serve as a shield to protect us from potential distress and may well be one of the most important ways to prevent stress.
        3. Close, rewarding relationships can provide a powerful emotional lift to boost your self-esteem and happiness and ultimately contribute to overall health and well-being.

II. **SOCIAL SUPPORT**
    A. **Social support** is the knowledge or belief by an individual that he or she is cared for and loved, belongs to a network of communication, and has a mutual obligation with others in the network.
        1. The social support system of an individual is made up of all the people who help meet financial, personal, physical, and emotional needs.
        2. Social support is belonging, being accepted, feeling loved, and being needed.
        3. The benefits of social support come not only from feeling supported, but also from our ability to give caring support to others.
    B. There are several different types of social support.
        1. **Instrumental or tangible support**, such as giving assistance through money, use of a car, or a place to stay.
        2. **Emotional support**, which consists of building esteem, emotional comfort, love, trust, concern, or listening.
        3. **Informational support**, which consists of giving advice, suggestions, directives, and information.
        4. **Appraisal support**, which provides affirmation, feedback, and information for self-evaluation.
    C. Social support provides a buffer for stress in a couple of ways.
        1. Support received at the point of appraisal of a potential threat.
        2. During the coping phase of a stressful situation when the person is trying to recover from the stressful experience.
    D. Social support has a positive effect on a person's health.
        1. An individual's health status and risk of dying were strongly associated with the extent and nature of his social network.
            a) This association remains true even after unhealthy behaviors were taken into consideration.
        2. In a study of breast cancer survivors, women who joined a support group after surgery lived twice as long as those who didn't.
        3. Married men live longer than single men.
        4. The effects of social support and stress on the immune system provide more evidence that a support system can help alleviate the major stress of poor health.
    E. Social support means having the support of people you trust and can talk to, to whom you feel a close connection, and with whom you share both the good times and the bad.
        1. Social support probably acts in part through its ability to buffer stress and protect a person from the diseases caused by stress.

III. **RELATIONSHIPS**
    A. Relationships play an important role in determining whether the young adult and college

        years are satisfying and positive or lonely and stressful.

    1.   Throughout life, the close relationships we develop and maintain shape who we become and how we deal with life.

B.   Stress often involves our relationships with other people.

    1.   We argue, fight, and worry when things aren't going right with the important people in our lives.

    2.   The way we interact with those around us can have a potent effect on the stress that we feel.

        a)   The relationships we have with others may even reflect the relationship we have with ourselves.

    3.   A full and rewarding social life can nourish the mind, the emotions, and the spirit, and good physical health depends as much on these aspects of our selves as it does on a strong and well-functioning body.

C.   Stress-relieving, loving relationships are not limited to humans.

    1.   Owning a pet, which constitutes a giving and receiving relationship, has long-term medical benefits.

        a)   Pet owners have longer lives and fewer stress symptoms than non-pet owners.

        b)   Pet therapy has been useful in dealing with emotional problems in people of all ages and situations.

    2.   Across the human lifespan, pets provide love and are a source of stress-relieving comfort.

D.   John Gottman found that conflict is common in relationships, but only 31 percent of conflicts get resolved over the course of a marriage.

    1.   The other 69 percent continue as unsolvable problems.

    2.   While disagreements and fights are not pleasant, they are necessary in some degree to all good marriages.

    3.   Couples who experience success in their marriage unions maintain the *five-to-one ratio*:

        a)   Stable relationships have five times as many positive factors, such as love, affection, interest in one another, humor, and support, as negative factors.

            (1) Maintaining a consistent balance of five loving or kind events for every instance of anger, contempt, or complaint keeps a marriage relationship healthy.

            (2) Success is based on a greater amount of positive factors than negative factors.

    4.   How a couple handles the inevitable differences that arise in any relationship is the key to their success or failure.

E.   People need to feel loved, and relationships are nurtured when we understand how to give and receive that love.

    1.   When this need is not met, the relationship will suffer no matter how committed the partnership.

        a)   Just as we need gas to keep our cars running, if people have empty love tanks they feel unloved, or unappreciated.

    2.   The key to a great relationship is figuring out what your partner needs in order to feel most loved, and then doing it.

    3.   People express love and receive love in different ways called Love Languages.

        a)   Words of Affirmation

        b)   Quality Time

        c)   Receiving Gifts

        d)   Acts of Service

        e)   Physical Touch

    4.   When people receive love in their preferred Love Language, they feel fulfilled.

    5.   Discovering and communicating with your partner in his or her preferred Love

Language can be facilitated by asking these questions:

    a) What does your partner do or fail to do that hurts you most deeply? The opposite of what hurts you most is probably your love language.

    b) What have you most often requested of your partner? The thing you have most often requested is likely the thing that would make you feel the most loved.

    c) In what way do you regularly express love to your partner? Your method of expressing love may be an indication of what would also make you feel loved.

6. It is important to pass this information on to the person with whom you have a deep relationship.

    a) If you don't let your partner know your preferred Love Language, chances are you won't get your love tank filled.

IV. COMMUNICATION

A. Relationships develop through communication.

B. One of the most important qualities for a relationship to survive and thrive is effective communication.

C. Communication between people is not always perfectly clear.

    1. The sender's message may not be delivered with the precise meaning that was intended.

    2. The person receiving the message does not always capture the precise meaning the sender meant to give.

D. Communication occurs from our earliest days and happens in many ways

    1. Speaking, reading, writing, observing, body language and listening are ways we communicate.

    2. Of these, listening may be the type of communication for which we receive the least amount of training.

E. Dr. Stephen Covey stated, "The single most important principle in the field of interpersonal relations is this: Seek first to understand, then to be understood. Most people listen, not with the intent to understand, but with the intent to reply."

    1. We tend to listen in the way that Covey calls **autobiographical listening**:

        a) We evaluate:

        b) We probe:

        c) We advise or tell

        d) We interpret

    2. The most advanced form of listening is called **empathic listening** - there are 4 stages to empathic listening:

        a) Stage 1 - Mimic content of communication

        b) Stage 2 - Rephrase the content

        c) Stage 3 - Reflect feeling

        d) Stage 4 - Reflect feeling

    3. Empathic listening is not appropriate in all circumstances.

        a) It is most effective when the interaction has a strong emotional component, when we are not sure that we understand and when we are not sure the other person feels confident that we understand.

        b) It is unnecessary to listen empathically when the conversation deals primarily with facts or logic.

        c) The moment responses become emotional, empathic listening is necessary.

    4. Tips for empathic listening

        a) Listen more, talk less.

        b) Suspend judgment.

        c) Look for the interesting aspects of the other person.

        d) Avoid giving advice.

        e) Allow moments of silence.

    f)   Listen with your eyes and your heart as much as your ears.
    g)   Use appropriate body signals.
F. Another form of non-verbal communication, we may communicate more with our touch than with our words.
    1.   Touch is one of the ultimate expressions of caring relationships.
        a)   A substantial body of research in both animals and humans supports the fact that caring touch is necessary for emotional health.
    2.   Through the sense of touch, messages from the external environment come to the attention of the body and mind.
        a)   Touch can make that message a positive one by reinforcing our perceived social support.
        b)   Do not underestimate touch as a powerful form of communication.
G. Men and Women - Different Can Be Good
    1.   When women are stressed they tend to feel a need to talk about their feelings.
        a)   Women may be less concerned with finding solutions than with feeling relief through expressing concerns and feeling understood.
    2.   In contrast, when men get upset they are less likely to talk about their concerns.
        a)   Men tend to think about the problem, mulling it over to find a solution.
        b)   If they can't find a solution, men are likely to do something to forget the problem.
    3.   Although Gray's idea about how men and women deal with stress and how they prefer to be treated when they are stressed is a generalization, the point that he makes is that people respond to love in different ways and if we don't treat them lovingly in the way that resonates with them, the loving gesture will not be seen as such.
        a)   People do not see things the same, nor do they require the same responses to feel listened to and supported.
        b)   The key is to respect and appreciate the differences in each person.

V. **MANAGING CONFLICT**
A. **Conflict** is an expressed struggle between at least two independent parties who perceive incompatible goals, scarce rewards, and interference from the other party in achieving their goals.
    1.   When the conflict can be described in a clear, concise way the parties stand a better chance of solving a problem before it becomes unsolvable or destructive.
        a)   Too often it is mistakenly believed that one individual understands exactly what the other person is thinking and feeling.
B. Conflict can be constructive.
    1.   Confronting disagreements through productive communication can lead to positive growth and improvement.
    2.   Frequently conflict is associated with stressful outcomes such as aggression, anger, damaged relationships, violence, and even wars. However, conflict is not an enemy.
        a)   Differences of opinions present an opportunity to consider solutions that would never be examined or explored. **Assertiveness** is constructive when dealing with conflict.
    3.   Different situations and different people require different techniques for resolving conflict.
C. While there is not a right or wrong style, it is helpful to rank either high or low the importance of the individual's needs or goals involved in the conflict, then apply the appropriate style of conflict resolution at the right time.
    1.   The Avoidance Style of Conflict Resolution (Turtle)
        a)   The avoidance style is unassertive and uncooperative.
        b)   Common characteristics of the turtle style of conflict management are these:

            (1) Non-confrontational

            (2) Denies issues that are a problem

            (3) Highly dependent person without inner direction

            (4) May postpone conflict or avoid it at all costs

            (5) Moves away, leaves, loses

    c) When to Use Avoidance

            (1) When the stakes aren't that high and you don't have anything to lose; when the issue is trivial.

            (2) When you don't have time to deal with it; when more important issues are pressing.

            (3) When the context isn't suitable; it isn't the right time or place.

            (4) When you see no chance of getting your concerns met.

            (5) When you would have to deal with an angry, hot-headed person.

            (6) When you are totally unprepared, taken by surprise, and you need time to think and collect information.

            (7) When you are too emotionally involved and the others around you can solve the conflict more successfully.

The Accommodating Style of Conflict Resolution (Teddy Bear)

    a) The Accommodating style is unassertive and cooperative.

    b) This is the opposite of competing.

    c) When accommodating, an individual neglects his own concerns to satisfy the concerns of the other person.

    d) There is an element of self-sacrifice in this mode.

    e) Common characteristics of the teddy bear of conflict management are these:

            (1) Agreeable, non-assertive

            (2) Cooperative even at expense of personal goals

            (3) Yielding; moves toward the other person; friendly

    f) When to Use Accommodating

            (1) When the issue is not so important to you but it is to the other person.

            (2) When maintaining the relationship outweighs other considerations.

            (3) When you discover that you are wrong.

            (4) When continued competition would be detrimental; you know you can't win.

            (5) When preserving harmony without disruption is most important; it's not the right time.

3. The Competing Style of Conflict Resolution (Shark)

    a) The competing style is aggressive and uncooperative.

    b) An individual pursues his or her own concerns at the other person's expense.

    c) This is a power-oriented mode in which one uses whatever power seems appropriate to win one's position.

    d) Common characteristics of the shark style of conflict management are these:

            (1) Uses power, position, personality or status to get own way

            (2) Academics, athletics, and the law commonly reflect this mindset

            (3) Assertive and aggressive

            (4) Forceful, moving against others

    e) When to Use Competition

            (1) When you know you are right.

            (2) When you need a quick decision.

            (3) When you meet a steamroller type of person and you need to stand

up for your own rights.

4. The Compromising Style of Conflict Resolution (Fox)
   a) Compromising is an intermediate position between assertiveness and cooperativeness.
   b) The objective of compromise is to find some expedient, mutually acceptable solution which partially satisfies both parties.
   c) Common characteristics of the fox style of conflict management are these:
     (1) Assertive but cooperative
     (2) Tries to bargain, compromise, and split the difference
   d) When to Use Compromising
     (1) When the goals are moderately important and not worth the use of more assertive modes.
     (2) When people of equal status are equally committed.
     (3) To reach temporary settlement on complex issues.
     (4) To reach expedient solutions on important issues.
     (5) As a back-up mode when competition or collaboration don't work.

5. The Collaborating Style of Conflict Resolution (Owl)
   a) The collaborating style is both assertive and cooperative.
   b) Collaboration involves an attempt to work with the other person to find some solution that fully satisfies the concerns of both persons.
   c) It includes identifying the underlying concerns of the two individuals and finding an alternative which meets both sets of concerns.
   d) The common term for this type of conflict resolution is win-win.
   e) This way of resolving conflicts is usually the most satisfying to all parties involved with the least amount of negative feelings.
   f) Common characteristics of the owl style of conflict management are these:
     (1) High respect for mutual benefit
     (2) Recognizes the needs and mutual benefit of both parties
     (3) Strives for win-win situation or recognizes abilities and expertise of all
     (4) Integrating; works toward solution with others
   g) When to Use Collaboration:
     (1) When other's lives are involved.
     (2) When you don't want to have full responsibility.
     (3) When there is a high level of trust.
     (4) When you want to gain commitment from others.
     (5) When you need to work through hard feelings or animosity.

D. Understanding the appropriate ways to resolve conflicts can make an enormous difference in the stress that we feel.
   1. Relationships invariably contain emotions that can run the gamut from ecstasy and joy to severe heartache and suffering.
   2. By practicing appropriate solutions to conflicts, we can remain on the more positive end of the emotional roller coaster that accompanies relationships.

VI. CONCLUSION
A. Social support is belonging, feeling accepted and loved, and being needed.
B. Our support systems are comprised of a web of relationships.
   1. From the moment we are born, bonding with our parents starts us down a path of personal relationships that shape our experience of trust and confidence in dealing with life.
   2. Having supportive, healthy relationships with other people can help protect against stress and are essential for physical, emotional, and social health.
C. Effective communication skills are essential for developing and maintaining relationships.

LEARNING ACTIVITIES

ACTIVITY 1 - JOURNALING

Objective: The purpose of this activity is to encourage critical thinking and honest personal reflection on topics relating to the chapter content. Explore personal thoughts, feelings, values, and behaviors as you selectively incorporate stress management knowledge and behaviors into your plan for improved health through better stress management.

Instructions: You will find journaling questions in each chapter of your Activities Manual. These questions relate specifically to the chapter content. Moving your thoughts from your mind to the paper is a powerful strategy for relieving stress and for increasing awareness of your thoughts, feelings and behaviors. Your course instructor can provide further guidance on how to complete this activity.

Complete the following journaling questions. Select the questions that have the most relevance for you.

1. Who do you turn to for support? Who do you support?
2. Think of a time when you have really needed supportive relationships to help you deal with a stressful time. What was it about the people that supported you that made their support so helpful to you?
3. What are your thoughts about the information from Gray's "Men Are from Mars, Women Are from Venus"? Think of an example based on your experience showing how men and women may communicate differently. What are some ways to bridge the gap?
4. How are your listening skills? Do you tend to be more of an empathic listener or an autobiographical listener? Ask someone who knows you well to honestly rate you. Try deliberately practicing empathic listening, and see how it turns out.
5. Do you feel comfortable being touched by others or are you a person who needs your "space" without the intrusion of others? What could you do to allow others to more fully communicate with you through touch?
6. Review the research on pets and the role they play in health. If you have a pet, how have you noticed the effect of your pet on your health? Have you had any personal experience demonstrating how a pet helped you deal with stress?
7. How does the information in this chapter affect you personally? What insights did you have about yourself and the stress that you experience?

ACTIVITY 2 – EMPATHIC LISTENING

Objectives: The purpose of this activity is to give you practice listening empathically.

Materials needed:
Handout 13:1 – Listening Empathically

Description of Activity: Complete Handout 13:1 – Listening Empathically. Use a listening opportunity where the other person has some emotional energy about something. Don't use empathic listening if they are talking about something mundane or an event that is not emotionally charged.

Handout 13:1 - Listening Empathically

Your assignment is to spend 30-45 minutes listening empathically to someone who is talking with you. You will listen to him or her according to the instructions for listening empathically in chapter 13 of your text. Talk with someone who is working with some issue that includes some emotional energy. You will not tell them that you are listening to them as an assignment. You will simply focus all of your listening energy on listening for the single purpose of understanding. After you have finished, respond to the following questions in a typed format.

1. Describe the situation: Who was involved? What was the main topic of conversation?
2. Describe how you noticed yourself vacillating between listening empathically and listening autobiographically.
3. Describe how the person you were talking with responded to you when you listened empathically.
4. Describe how easy or difficult you found that it was to listen empathically for that long.

Be thorough with your responses.

ACTIVITY 3 - HAPPY RELATIONSHIPS

Objective: The purpose of this activity is to increase your awareness of factors that contribute to a happy relationship.

Instructions: Interview a couple who have been married or been partners for more than 25 years. Ask the couple for the top five things that they think contributes to a successful, happy relationship. Bring your list to class and compile a master list of responses. Discuss how these findings relate to stress. You might notice differences between men's responses and women's responses.

An interesting adaptation of this activity is to interview each of the partners separately and then bring them together to share the results. This can lead to some discussion on similarities and differences in their perceptions of what contributes to a fulfilling relationship.

ACTIVITY 4 - DISCOVERING YOUR "LOVE LANGUAGE"

Objectives: The purpose of this activity is to help you determine your preferred Love Language according to the information in chapter 13.

Materials needed: Blank piece of paper and pen or pencil

Description of Activity: This activity can be done individually or in pairs. If in pairs, one will go first and the other will serve as a support and guide.

Think back to a time in your life when you felt deeply loved. Try as much as possible to relive the situation in your mind. If you aren't able to picture it clearly, simply sense the situation and how you were feeling.

Once you are sure you have in mind the loving situation, try to observe what was happening that made you feel loved. Were you being touched in a certain way? Were you being told you were loved in certain ways? Were other people doing things for you? Were you spending quality time with someone else? Because of being given things did you feel loved?

Based on what you observed, identify your primary love language.

Additional questions to consider in determining your love language include:

1. What does your partner do or fail to do that hurts you most deeply? The opposite of what hurts you most is probably your love language.
2. What have you most often requested of your partner? The thing you have requested most often is likely the thing that would make you feel the most loved.
3. In what way do you express love to your partner regularly? Your method of expressing love may be an indication of what also would make *you* feel loved.

ACTIVITY 5 - TRUST WALK

Objectives: The purpose of this activity is to give you the opportunity to develop your sense of trust in another person.

Materials needed:
Handout 13:2 - Trust Walk Thoughts
Blindfolds

Description of Activity: Follow the directions given by your teacher for this in-class activity. Complete Handout 13:2.

Handout 13:2 - Trust Walk Thoughts

Name _____

Thoroughly respond to each question:

1. What was your experience of the Trust Walk when you were blindfolded? (Include thoughts, feelings, etc.)

2. What was your experience of the Trust Walk when you were the guide? (Include thoughts, feelings, etc.)

3. What aspects of the walk made you uncomfortable or did you find fearful? How did you find yourself dealing with them?

4. What aspects of the walk did you feel promoted positive thoughts and feelings?

RELATED WEBSITES

Empathy and Listening Skills for Emotional Intimacy
A website that discusses empathy, listening skills, and acknowledgments, and their effects on the emotional intimacy of two people involved in a conversation.
http://www.touch-another-heart.com/

Keep Love Alive
An interview with Leo Buscaglia
http://www.intouchmag.com/interview.html

Social Support: Why and How
A discussion by Dr. David Posen on the effect of social support on stress
http://www.davidposen.com/pages/tips/tips20.html

CHAPTER 14
CREATING A HEALING ENVIRONMENT

CHAPTER OUTLINE

Use this outline to take notes as you read the chapter in the text and/or as your instructor lectures in class.

I. CREATING A HEALING ENVIRONMENT
    A. How does environment affect stress and what can we do about it?

II. STRESS AND THE ENVIRONMENT
    A. **Environment** includes everything both internal and external to an individual.
    B. An **environmental stressor** is some aspect of our environment that is perceived as annoying, distracting, uncomfortable, or stressful. The following can be considered environmental stressors:
        1. Air pollution
        2. Noise
        3. Overcrowding
        4. Disasters (natural and manmade)
        5. Climate conditions
        6. Lighting
        7. Colors of a room
        8. Insects
        9. Tobacco smoke
        10. Poor ergonomics
        11. The arrangement of furniture
        12. Room clutter
        13. Room temperature.
    C. Individual perceptions play a part in the stress that we feel in a given environment.
        1. There is strong agreement that the physical environment impacts how we think, feel, and act.
        2. Like all stressors, environmental stressors are different for each of us.
            a) One person may perceive going to a rock concert and sitting in front of the speakers as pleasurable and relaxing.
            b) To another person, this would be one of the most stressful experiences imaginable.
        3. Perception is the important component of whether an environmental factor is stressful.
    D. **Learned response theory** helps explain why we might feel stressed in certain environments.
        1. Sometimes perception is based on past experience.
        2. When we associate a particular environment with something painful in that environment, the two get linked together.
        3. The result can be that we perceive the environment itself as unpleasant.
            a) Simply being in an environment associated in our mind with discomfort or pain can elicit the stress response even when there is no pain or danger.
                (1) An example of this might be a woman who experiences morning sickness during the early stages of her pregnancy and also spends time shopping in a particular shopping mall.
                (2) Repeated exposure to the mall combined with her morning sickness may trigger the unpleasant response of feeling sick each time she goes to the mall in the future after the pregnancy is over.
                (3) A shopping mall would not, under normal conditions, cause this response, but when one condition is paired with another, and pain or discomfort is involved, the environment becomes a trigger for this response.

III. MANAGING ENVIRONMENTAL STRESSORS
    A. Many people do not even notice the effects the environment has on them.

1. They become accustomed to living and working in environments that are not, by their nature, natural, pleasant, and peaceful
   a) This disconnection from the natural world can leave people feeling estranged and unfulfilled. They may feel stressed and seek artificial substitutes for natural experiences.

B. By taking a proactive approach toward environmental stressors, you may be able to reduce or eliminate stressors from your environment.
1. If you can't eliminate the stressor, try to remove yourself from the environment or try to adapt and think differently so the stressor isn't perceived as painful or uncomfortable.
   a) Some stressors in the environment are not in our control.
2. The creation of a calming, healing environment in our home and surroundings is usually within our control.

IV. A HEALING ENVIRONMENT
A. A **healing environment** is one in which individuals are supported and nurtured, in which they feel calm, and in which health and well-being are promoted.
1. Healing environments may be just as important as eating properly, exercising regularly, practicing proper health care, and having meaningful relationships and support systems.

V. COLOR
A. Colors can raise or lower your stress and energy level.
1. Color affects heart rates, brainwave activity, respirations, and muscle tension.
2. Color has meaning to most people, and lack of color can be a source of stress.
3. Color can make a space feel restful, cheerful, stimulating, or irritating.
4. **Chromotherapy** is a discipline that uses colors to treat individuals suffering from certain disorders.
   a) Warmer colors such as peach, soft yellows or coral can stimulate the appetite and encourage alertness, creativity, and socialization; these colors are useful in such areas as dining rooms or meeting spaces.
   b) Blues, greens, violets, and other cool colors are useful in areas designed to be restful, spiritual, contemplative, and quiet, such as bedrooms or meditation areas.
   c) Primary colors - red, yellow, and blue - and strong patterns are pleasing at first but can be overstimulating and may contribute to fatigue.
   d) Green symbolizes growth, healing, spirituality, and peace, and has been used to reduce tension and nervousness.
   e) The brain requires constant stimulation. Monotonous color schemes contribute to sensory deprivation, disorganization of brain function, deterioration of intelligence, and an inability to concentrate. They slow the healing process and are perceived as "institutional."
   f) Color affects an individual's perception of time, size, weight, and volume. For example, warm color schemes are better in rooms where pleasant activities, such as dining or recreation, take place, since the activity seems to last longer. In rooms where monotonous tasks are performed, a cool color scheme can make time pass more quickly.

VI. LIGHT
A. Light is a form of electromagnetic energy that can have both positive and negative effects on living organisms.
1. The importance of natural sunlight to healing has been explored in a number of strong studies including the following:
   a) Depressed patients in a psychiatric unit recovered faster in rooms with brighter lights.
   b) Increased exposure to daylight was found to have a uniformly positive and statistically significant effect on student performance as evidenced by better test scores.
   c) Increased daytime light exposure had an impact on nighttime sleep quality

in both hospitalized and healthy youth.

2. Shorter periods of daylight, as occur naturally in the winter, have been shown to trigger **seasonal affective disorder** (SAD).
   a) SAD is a mood disorder associated with depression episodes and related to seasonal variations of light.
   b) Symptoms include depression, irritability, and fatigue.
   c) Regular exposure to full-spectrum lighting has been demonstrated to improve SAD by increasing the amount of **melatonin** produced by the **pineal gland**.
3. Natural daylight is believed to be best for health, yet many people live and work in environments lit by fluorescent lighting.
   a) Full-spectrum fluorescent lamps have been designed as an alternative to traditional fluorescent lighting.
      (1) They mimic the spectral qualities of daylight and provide similar health-promoting effects to those of natural light.

VII. **SMELLS AND AIR**
A. Smell can play a role in managing stress.
   1. Smell is analyzed in the limbic part of the brain, an area associated with emotions.
      a) It is not surprising then that an aroma can affect how we feel.
   2. **Aromatherapy**, the therapeutic use of essential oils, can lower stress levels.
      a) Smelling the essential oils can send a direct message to your brain via your olfactory nerves, where they can then affect the endocrine and hormonal systems via the hypothalamus.
      b) Odors have the effect on our emotional states because they hook into the emotional or primitive parts of our brains such as the limbic system.
      c) Certain essential oils from plants and flowers, such as lavender, rose, neroli, and petitgrain, are well known for this ability.
         (1) Jasmine and rosemary have been found to increase beta waves in the brain and result in a more alert state, while lavender increases the brain's alpha waves, thus promoting relaxation.
   3. Air Quality - A good deep breath of fresh air can clear the mind and calm the body.

VIII. **NOISE**
A. We are surrounded by hundreds of potentially stressful sounds every day.
   1. Noise from machinery and industrial plants; road, rail, and air traffic; business and community services; construction; domestic activities; and leisure activities make noise one of our most pervasive pollutants.
   2. We have all experienced stress from noise, whether it be the TV blaring while you are trying to read, the non-stop talker sitting next to you in the library, your neighbor mowing his yard while you are trying to nap in the hammock, or the party going on next door while you are trying to sleep.
      a) Noise is measured in **decibels**. If you must be exposed to louder noises, it is recommended that you limit the exposure time and/or wear hearing protection.
   3. **Perceived noisiness** describes the subjective assessment of noise that combines the decibel level and the context in which a noise occurs.
      a) What is noise to one person can be appreciated sound to another.
      b) Noise becomes a stressor when we appraise it as annoying or subjectively determine it to be stressful because it interferes with our ability to concentrate, function, or relax.
B. Environmental noise is related to stress levels
   1. Many studies have linked noise exposure to increased health risk and decreased well-being.
      a) Noise can fray the nerves.
         (1) People tend to be more anxious, irritable, and angry when their ears are constantly barraged with sound. Researchers speculate that noise, especially if it stresses the mother, may even be

hazardous to their unborn babies.

2. Relaxing sounds such as **white noise** in the form of nature sounds, widely available for purchase, helps to drown out other sounds that may be distracting and stressful.
    a) Studies show that the sounds of running water and relaxing music can stimulate the production of endorphins and lower heart rates.

IX. TEMPERATURE

A. The **heat hypothesis** states that hot temperatures can increase aggressive motives and behaviors.
    1. The **heat effect** describes higher rates of aggression in people who are hot relative to people who are cooler.
    2. Hot temperatures increase aggression by directly increasing feelings of hostility and indirectly increasing aggressive thoughts.
        a) Better climate controls in many institutional settings, like prisons, schools, and workplaces, may reduce stress and tension and the resulting aggression-related problems.
    3. Heat-induced discomfort makes people cranky and lowers their tolerance level resulting in feelings of anger.

X. AESTHETIC QUALITY OF SURROUNDINGS

A. **Feng shui** (pronounced "phung schway") is the ancient Chinese study of the natural environment.
    1. It is based on the belief that physical and emotional well-being is strongly influenced by our immediate environment.
    2. Practitioners of feng shui use a special compass, called a **lo-pan**, to determine the energy characteristics of a building or room.
    3. The layout of spaces and arrangement of furniture is said to affect the energy flow.
        a) The idea is to balance the energy so it will have a positive effect.
        b) Good **chi**, or energy flow, is believed to have a strong impact on the health and peace of mind of occupants.
    4. Feng shui consultants guide architects in positioning and arranging buildings such as hospitals, offices, and the rooms within the buildings.
    5. Interior designers apply the principles in the arrangement of furniture, the use of plants and other living things, the placement of mirrors and pictures, and the choice of colors.
B. Human beings are intimately connected to nature.
    1. They share the planet with every other living organism and they are just one strand in the complex web of life.
    2. When they live a disconnected existence, they become unhealthy, unbalanced, and unhappy.
    3. Yet, when they are in a healing environment, they know it. They feel welcome, balanced, relaxed, reassured, and stimulated.
    4. You may not be able to get outdoors a lot, but you can do a few things to increase the amount of nature in your current environment.
        a) Indoor and outdoor gardens
        b) Bring nature indoors
        c) Arrange your home and office to get maximum enjoyment from the view of nature
        d) Artwork of relaxing nature scenes
        e) Light and fresh air
C. Organize and Simplify
    1. Creating a simple, uncluttered environment can reduce your stress.
    2. Eliminate the useless clutter in your life.

XI. ERGONOMICS

A. **Ergonomics** is the study of individual workers and the tasks they perform for the purpose of designing appropriate living and working environments.
B. The major goals of ergonomics are to make work safer and enhance worker and worksite

well-being.

       1. Much of the ergonomic research can also be applied to the home environment.

XII. TECHNOLOGY AND THE ENVIRONMENT

A. The impact that technology has on our environment is becoming increasingly significant.

    1. It is hard to imagine a world without computers.

    2. Computers and other technology have introduced new sources and symptoms of stress we could not have imagined a few years ago.

    3. Technology keeps coming at us and we are told that we must adapt or fall behind.

        a) No wonder 85 percent of us are hesitant or outright resistant to technology!

B. **Technostress** is the feeling of dependence, incompetence, anxiety, and frustration associated with our experience with technology. **Technosis** describes when a person becomes so immersed in technology that they risk losing their own identity.

    1. The growing dependence on technology can affect us negatively.

        a) We count on our machines to do so much that when something goes wrong with our technology we are thrown into a tailspin.

C. Several issue relate to how technology may contribute to a stressful environment:

    1. Alienation and isolation of people from each other.

    2. Blurring of the boundaries between work and home from the intrusion of computers and technology.

    3. Information overload and multi-tasking madness result in feeling overwhelmed.

    4. Higher expectations as computers and constantly changing software create demands for more efficiency and expectations of higher productivity.

    5. Pressure to keep up with "mine's bigger than yours."

    6. A pro-humanity, rather than an anti-technology, approach can encourage us to move forward with an uplifting, inspiring look at ways to master the Information Age.

        a) Some suggestions to help us perform better at work, spend more quality time with our families, and experience the wonder of technology without the technostress include the following:

           (1) Recognize that there is more technology than you will ever want or be able to use. With technology, like magazine subscriptions, you get to select what you want and only use what works for you. It's okay to leave the rest alone.

           (2) Understand that the way technology is implemented in most businesses practically guarantees technostress. In their "12-phase people-centric training model," Weil and Rosen encourage corporations to provide ample time for "free play" with any new technology to ensure success.

           (3) Just because technology is capable of doing multiple jobs at the same time does not mean that we are. "Multi-tasking madness" is hitting us all as we attempt to juggle more and more. It is interfering with our sleep at night and our concentration and memory by day.

           (4) At home, family members are in their own "techno-cocoons," each hooked up to a different techno-gadget. Create family rules for technological use to avoid this isolating trend.

XIII. CONCLUSION

A. Many aspects of your surroundings can contribute to a relaxing, stress-reducing environment.

    1. Think about how you can use color, noise, smells, light, and nature to create a healing environment.

    2. Think about how you manage technology.

    3. Create an environment that contributes to your sense of peace and control in a sometimes chaotic world.

    4. The peace you create at home will spread to our communities and beyond.

4. LEARNING ACTIVITIES

ACTIVITY 1 - JOURNALING

Objective: The purpose of this activity is to encourage critical thinking and honest personal reflection on topics relating to the chapter content. Explore personal thoughts, feelings, values, and behaviors as you selectively incorporate stress management knowledge and behaviors into your plan for improved health through better stress management.

Instructions: You will find journaling questions in each chapter of your Activities Manual. These questions relate specifically to the chapter content. Moving your thoughts from your mind to the paper is a powerful strategy for relieving stress and for increasing awareness of your thoughts, feelings and behaviors. Your course instructor can provide further guidance on how to complete this activity.

Complete the following journaling questions. Select the questions that have the most relevance for you.

1. Are there environments in which you feel stressed? Think about places where you might feel more stressed. Discuss what it is about the environment that may be contributing to your stress
2. Of all the environmental factors discussed in this chapter what are the two or three that can contribute the most to creating a more peaceful environment for you? Discuss one specific thing that you will do to make your environment more relaxing.
3. Do some research on feng shui. Do you believe the idea of energy flow in a room or building is credible? Do you think this flow of energy could contribute to positive feelings? If so, how?
4. Discuss your results on the technosis quiz. Evaluate your use of technology from the perspective of how it makes your life more enjoyable. Ask someone who knows you to give their impression of how you use technology.
5. How does the information in this chapter affect you personally? What insights did you have about yourself and the stress that you experience?

ACTIVITY 2 - HOW HEALING IS YOUR ENVIRONMENT?

Objective: The purpose of this activity is to increase your awareness of your environment.

Instructions: Conduct an evaluation of your environment using Handout 14:1. You can choose any setting such as your dorm room, home, the student union, campus library, or even a classroom in which you spend a lot of time. Complete the worksheet and bring it to class.

HANDOUT 14:1 – HOW HEALING IS YOUR ENVIRONMENT?

Name: _____

Directions: Complete this worksheet on a place where you spend considerable time. You could choose your dorm room, the library, your home, the student union, or even a classroom.

Location you are assessing:

Describe the environment in as much detail as possible including color, light, smells, air, noise, and temperature. Also include the aesthetic quality of the setting as described in your textbook.

What aspects of the environment do you find to be relaxing? Why?

What aspects of the environment do you find to be stressful? Why?

What are three things you would or could do to make this environment more relaxing and healing?

ACTIVITY 3 - ASSESSING A WEB SITE

Objective: The purpose of this activity is to provide you with an opportunity to explore and critique a website related to the environment.

Instructions: Explore either one of the websites listed in this chapter or a different website related to the environment. Type up a brief summary of the website including what you learned from viewing this site and whether or not you would recommend this site to another and why. Include a brief critique of the site.

RELATED WEBSITES

Technostress
Just as fat has replaced starvation as this nation's number one dietary concern, information overload has replaced information scarcity as an important new emotional, social, and political problem. This website gives ideas for dealing with technostress.
http://www.virtualcs.com/nmhi/lesson7_1.html

Feng Shui Ultimate Resource
Website designed to help Feng Shui shed its snake-oil-and-incense image
http://www.qi-whiz.com/

Aromatherapy
This site presents excellent information on all aspects of aromatherapy
http://www.aromaweb.com/

CHAPTER 15
HEALTHY LIFESTYLES

<u>CHAPTER OUTLINE</u>
Use this outline to take notes as you read the chapter in the text and/or as your instructor lectures in class.

I. **HEALTHY LIFESTYLES**
    A. Stress is known to influence health not only through its direct physiological effect, but also through its indirect effect via altered health behaviors.
    B. Maintaining a healthy lifestyle includes avoiding activities that people sometimes believe will help them relax or cope with the stress that they feel.
    C. Taking care of your body is an important strategy for preventing stress.
    D. A strong, healthy body is more resilient, more able to adapt, and less likely to experience the negative effects of stress at the mental, emotional, physical, social, and spiritual levels.

II. **EXERCISE**
    A. Exercise is one of our most powerful stress buffers for a variety of reasons.
    B. Nothing has been found to be as generally beneficial for health and well-being as regular physical activity or exercise.
    C. To understand why exercise is beneficial in buffering stress, recall the earlier discussions in Chapter 3 about the stress response.
        1. The stress response occurs when we sense the need to either run from or fight a potential threat.
            a) When we sense danger, the body automatically gears up for activity, namely running or fighting.
            b) Therefore, it eases stress to follow through on that message and participate in activities that use our fighting and running muscles - exercise.
            c) By participating in activities that use our fighting and running muscles, the body uses excess blood sugar; muscles use the stress hormones adrenaline and cortisol; and other circulating fats in the bloodstream get used for energy.
            d) During exercise, the body goes through a process similar to the stress response; that is, there is a period of arousal and hyperstimulation followed by a period of exhaustion and rest.
    D. Other Benefits of Exercise
        1. Exercise generates the natural release of the mood-lifting hormones called endorphins from the brain.
            a) These "feel-good" hormones act the same way the chemical morphine acts in the body, only without the negative side effects.
        2. Exercise can also give you a sense of accomplishment and boost your confidence.
        3. Exercise increases the flow of blood to the brain, improving concentration and alertness, helping you to think more clearly.
        4. Physical conditioning also offers important protection.
            a) The person whose heart, lungs, and skeletal muscles are conditioned by exercise can withstand cardiovascular and respiratory effects of the alarm stage of stress better than someone who leads a sedentary life.
        5. Because exercise relieves stress, a physically fit person does not get sick as often due to a healthy functioning immune system.
        6. A physically fit person gets injured less frequently and has greater endurance, and as a result would be less likely to feel as fatigued at the end of a long day.
            a) When we work out, we are participating in an activity over which we usually have total control.

    E. For optimal results, exercise should be regular and balance the following components of physical fitness.

        1. Cardiorespiratory fitness

        2. Muscle fitness, muscle strength, and **muscle endurance**

        3. Flexibility

        4. Body Composition

    F. The best type of exercise is the one you will do.

        1. Equally important is what you want to accomplish from your exercise.

            a) Refer to Table 15-1 for the right type of exercise depending on the mood you are in.

    G. Three things help people start and stick with an exercise routine:

        1. Enjoyment

        2. Convenience

        3. Social Support.

III. NUTRITION

    A. Stress can initiate a wide variety of altered eating behaviors and create some unique nutritional needs.

    B. The best nutritional preparation for stress is a varied and balanced diet. The ***Dietary Guidelines for Americans*** provides science-based advice to promote health and reduce the risk of disease.

        1. Nutrition experts recommend a foundation of fresh fruits, fresh vegetables, whole grains, and legumes.

            a) Complex carbohydrates are an ideal anti-stress food because they boost the brain's level of the mood-enhancing chemical **serotonin**.

        2. Moderate amounts of protein and dairy foods are also included in a healthy diet.

        3. Whole grains are important to a healthy diet in part because of how they relate to blood sugar levels.

            a) Foods that enter the bloodstream quickly have a higher **glycemic index**.

                (1) The result of high glycemic index foods, like simple sugars, is that the blood sugar level increases rapidly.

                (2) The body responds by secreting insulin, which results in a decline of the blood sugar level.

                (3) This fluctuation can leave you feeling low on energy and less able to mentally and physically combat stress.

            b) Lower glycemic index foods, like whole grains, result in a more stable blood sugar level and as a result, a more stable mood and energy level.

    C. Low water levels in the body can dramatically affect our moods and perceptions.

        1. A decrease of as little as 1 to 3 percent in the body's water level can make us feel agitated and irritable.

        2. A 3 to 5 percent drop can lead to headaches, weakness, and fatigue.

        3. A drop of more than 5 percent can lead to hospitalization.

        4. Nutritionists recommend drinking enough water so that your urine is very light yellow or clear, not dark in color.

    D. For optimum health and stress management, limit your intake of caffeine, fats, sugars, and especially soft drinks.

        1. Excessive caffeine in your diet can lead to feelings of restlessness or nervousness (the "jitters") as well as a racing heartbeat, tremors, sleep disturbances, and nausea.

            a) Gradually reduce or eliminate the amount of caffeine you consume in a day.

        2. Foods that contain hydrogenated or partially hydrogenated oil, trans fatty acids, should be avoided as much as possible.

            a) Consumption of these and saturated fats results in an increase of plaque deposits in blood vessels which can lead to blood vessel diseases including heart disease and stroke.

    3. Soft Drinks contain about 12 teaspoons of sugar and often contain caffeine and other substances that are of no nutritional value to the body.

        a) Soft drinks have a high glycemic index.

    4. The carbonation in soft drinks also tends to inhibit mineral absorption.

E. Digesting food requires more energy than any other process in the body besides exercise.

    1. It's no wonder we are tired after eating a large, heavy meal.

IV. STRESS AND HEALTHY WEIGHT

A. Overeating, probably more than anything else, leads to the growing epidemic of overweight and obesity in our country. This is a source of great stress.

B. Emotional eating is often done without thinking about it and unrelated to hunger.

    1. There may be a connection between eating certain foods and the release of substances in the brain that are experienced as soothing.

    2. When we eat, our body releases a chemical called **dopamine** which makes us feel good and can help offset the pain that we may be feeling from our stressful day.

C. When the body experiences the fight-or-flight response, glucose is drawn from stored glycogen and fat.

    1. When glucose is not used for physical activity, as happens when we sense a threat but aren't in any danger, it is stored as fat.

D. Activation of the stress response results in massive secretion of the stress hormone cortisol.

    1. One of the jobs of cortisol is to store energy.

    2. The body knows that when it encounters threatening circumstances, there is the possibility that food may not be available in the near future, and stores energy as fat.

V. EATING DISORDERS

A. Eating disorders such as **anorexia**, **bulimia**, and **binge eating** include extreme emotions, attitudes, and behaviors surrounding weight and food issues.

    1. Research has highlighted the association between perceived stress and eating disorders such as binge eating.

    2. **Runaway eating** is the consistent use of food and food-related behaviors--such as purging or exercising excessively--to deal with unpleasant feelings and the sense that these feelings are out of control.

B. Eating disorders are complex conditions that arise from a combination of long-standing behavioral, emotional, psychological, interpersonal, and social factors.

    1. People with eating disorders often use food and the control of food in an attempt to compensate for feelings and emotions that may otherwise seem overwhelming.

    2. Dieting, bingeing, and purging may begin as a way to cope with painful emotions and to feel in control of one's life.

    3. Ultimately, these behaviors will damage a person's physical and emotional health, self-esteem, and sense of competence and control.

VI. SLEEP

A. Insufficient sleep is a prominent stressor and is responsible for a host of problems.

    1. Some people find it difficult to go to sleep quickly while others have difficulty staying asleep during the night.

    2. A good night's sleep is one in which your head hits the pillow, within a few minutes you are fast asleep, and the next thing you know it is morning and you wake up feeling refreshed and alert.

B. Stress and sleep affect each other.

    1. Stress is often a contributing factor to sleep problems and insufficient sleep contributes to stress.

C. There is no right amount of sleep for everyone.

    1. Some people function fine with six hours of sleep

    2. Others can't function optimally with less than nine.

    3. Most people need seven to eight hours of sleep per night.

D. Follow these suggestions for improving your sleep habits:
1. Go to bed at the same time each day.
2. Get up at the same time each day.
3. Get regular exercise each day. There is evidence that regular exercise improves restful sleep. This includes stretching and aerobic exercise.
4. Get regular exposure to outdoor or bright lights, especially in the late afternoon.
5. Keep the temperature in your bedroom comfortably cool. Have extra blankets if you get too cold.
6. Keep the bedroom quiet when sleeping.
7. Keep the bedroom dark enough to facilitate sleep.
8. Use your bed only for sleep and sex.
9. Try a relaxation exercise just before going to sleep.
10. Start winding down two hours before bedtime. This period of time allows the brain to wind down and decrease its activity so the sleep systems can take over.

E. Avoid these activities for improving sleep:
1. Consume caffeine in the evening (coffee, many teas, chocolate, and sodas).
2. Watch television in bed.
3. Use alcohol to help you sleep.
4. Go to bed too hungry or too full.
5. Take another person's sleeping pills.
6. Take over-the-counter sleeping pills without your doctor's knowledge. Tolerance can develop rapidly with some medications.
7. Try to force yourself to sleep. This only makes your mind and body more alert.
8. Sleep with your pets or children.
9. If you lie in bed awake for more than twenty to thirty minutes, get up and go to a different room, participate in a quiet activity, like reading, then return to bed when you feel sleepy.

VII. **LIFESTYLE BEHAVIORS TO AVOID**
A. In our culture, cigarettes are a common but questionable choice for combating stress.
1. Many smokers justify smoking as a means of dealing with their stress.
   a) Nicotine is a dangerous and addictive stimulant.
      (1) The effects of nicotine mimic that of the stress response in many ways
   b) There are many reasons why people choose to smoke as a way to cope with stress, but it will always be in the category of unhealthy and ineffective ways to manage stress because of the harmful long-term effects of smoking.

B. Alcohol is sometimes used as a form of self-medication to temporarily ease feelings of pain or stress.
1. Stress-related drinking is common especially in competitive academic environments where students turn to alcohol to reduce their anxiety and pressure to perform.
2. Many factors determine whether an individual will turn to alcohol as a means of coping with life's challenges.
   a) Whether an individual will drink in response to stress appears to depend on many factors, including possible genetic determinants, an individual's usual drinking behavior, one's expectations regarding the effect of alcohol on stress, the intensity and type of stressor, the individual's sense of control over the stressor, the range of one's responses to cope with the perceived stress, and the availability of social support to buffer the effects of stress.
3. More than one or two drinks per day can lead to many problems including alcoholism, liver diseases, various cancers, and many types of accidents.
   a) Drinking is also associated with other unhealthy behaviors such as smoking, sexual aggression, and violence.

C. Illegal drugs are unhealthy and ineffective for reducing stress.

       1. The results can be deceptive since some drugs create a cycle of dependency by masking the symptoms of stress, resulting in temporarily feeling better.

VIII.   **PUTTING IT ALL TOGETHER**

    A. Understanding that making healthy choices and living a healthy lifestyle is necessary for well-being is not a new idea to most of us, however it is an idea we need to be reminded of frequently.

        1. The key is that there is a difference between knowing and doing.

        2. Take time to carefully reflect on your daily choices.

            a) Focus on awareness of both the healthy and unhealthy ways that you choose to deal with stress.

            b) Decide how you can integrate more healthy choices into your routine and eliminate unhealthy choices.

IX. **CONCLUSION**

    A. Taking care of yourself through exercise, eating right, adequate sleep, and avoiding unhealthy behaviors is the foundation for good health.

LEARNING ACTIVITIES

ACTIVITY 1 - JOURNALING

Objective: The purpose of this activity is to encourage critical thinking and honest personal reflection on topics relating to the chapter content. Explore personal thoughts, feelings, values, and behaviors as you selectively incorporate stress management knowledge and behaviors into your plan for improved health through better stress management.

Instructions: You will find journaling questions in each chapter of your Activities Manual. These questions relate specifically to the chapter content. Moving your thoughts from your mind to the paper is a powerful strategy for relieving stress and for increasing awareness of your thoughts, feelings and behaviors. Your course instructor can provide further guidance on how to complete this activity.

Complete the following journaling questions. Select the questions that have the most relevance for you.

1. What would your ideal exercise program look like? Which kinds of exercise and activities do you enjoy the most? How can you incorporate these into your daily life?
2. Looking at the section in chapter 15 called "What Type of Exercise is Best?" which type of activity would probably be best for you to help you feel better than you do right now?
3. How does stress affect your eating habits and possible excess fat gain?
4. Think about these questions in relation to your current sleeping habits: How much sleep are you getting? What is the quality of your sleep? Do you feel refreshed and rested when you awaken in the morning? Do you feel you need more? Could you go to sleep earlier in the evening to help you get in more sleep?
5. Do you use or consider using alcohol as a way of coping with stress? What are the positive and negatives of using alcohol for coping with stress?
6. How does the information in this chapter affect you personally? What insights did you have about yourself and the stress that you experience?

ACTIVITY 2 - RELAXATION EXERCISE - GUIDED IMAGERY - FLOATING THROUGH COLORS

Objectives: The purpose of this activity is to allow you to practice deep relaxation on your own using the Guided Imagery - Floating through Colors relaxation exercise that is found on the Stress Relief DVD.

Materials needed:
Stress Relief DVD
Handout 15:1 - DVD Relaxation Exercise - Guided Imagery - Floating through Colors

Instructions:
1. Practice Guided Imagery - Floating through Colors at least two times on your own.

2. Complete Handout 15:1 - DVD Relaxation Exercise - Guided Imagery - Floating through Colors to help you assess your experience.

Handout 15:1 - DVD Relaxation Exercise
Guided Imagery - Floating through Colors

The DVD assignment for this week is the seventh exercise on the DVD called "Floating through Colors."
Do not do the other two guided imageries - Mountain Lake or Inner Wisdom - for this week's assignment!

Practice doing this exercise at least two (2) times according to the instructions on the DVD. Resist the urge to fall asleep, so ***don't*** do it just before you go to bed.

Do it at times when you will not be disturbed. It lasts approximately 15 minutes.

In a *typed* format, respond to the following items:

1. How you felt before the exercise
2. Your experience during the exercise
3. How you felt immediately following the exercise
4. How you felt long after completing the exercise

On your typed paper, ***thoroughly*** respond to each of these items referring to the two times that you did them at home, *and* the time that you did it in class. Describe primarily how you were feeling in relation to your stress levels.

Follow this general outline with your description:

Daytime (first time):
• Before
• During
• Immediately after
• Long after

Daytime (second time):
• Before
• During
• Immediately after
• Long after

Classroom experience (if applicable):
• Before
• During
• Immediately after
• Long after

ACTIVITY 3 - DISCOVERING YOUR SLEEP NEEDS

Objectives: The purpose of this activity is to show you how to determine how much sleep you need at night.

Instructions: There is no correct amount of sleep that a person should get each night. Most experts agree that about 7-9 hours of sleep is optimum, but this doesn't necessarily apply to everyone.

Follow these instructions to find out what your sleep needs are.

1. Try to go to sleep at the same time every night for 4 or 5 nights in a row.
2. Awaken in the morning without an alarm (this may not be possible until a break or summer vacation.)
3. Look at the clock upon awakening and calculate the hours that you slept.
4. Do the same for each of the 4 or five nights.
5. Add up all of the time that you spent sleeping and divide by the number of nights considered. This will give you an average amount of time. This average is a pretty good measure of your sleep needs.

Be sure to participate in typical activity (exercise) and eat at nearly the same times each of the days being considered in order to get an accurate assessment.

Note: Obviously sleep needs change depending on a variety of factors including activity levels, nutritional activity, stress levels, and even extreme mental activity (heavy-duty studying may require more rest to help the mind process what's been learned). Be sure to take these factors into account when you are looking at how much sleep you need.

ACTIVITY 4 - THE POWER OF EXERCISE TO REDUCE STRESS

Objectives: The purpose of this activity is to help you see the benefits of exercise toward reducing stress and as part of a healthy lifestyle.

Instructions: If possible, do this activity at a time when you are feeling very high levels of stress such as just before or after a huge test or after you've been in a heated argument with someone.

During this time of extreme stress, instead of watching TV or just sitting and thinking about the stressor, put on your running or workout shoes and go for a long jog, or go play racquetball and for about an hour just hit the ball as hard as you can (fortunately, in a racquetball court you can hit the ball as hard as you want and you won't have to chase it very far). Do something with enough intensity that you get out of breath and find yourself sweating for a while.

After you are finished, notice the change in how you feel. Certainly, the stressor hasn't changed, but you have followed through on the message you have been giving yourself to fight or run (fight-or-flight response) and you can now approach the situation in a more relaxed way.

Review Handout 15:2, Exercise Guidelines for Health-Related Physical Fitness. Think about the types and benefits of exercise and the importance of including regular exercise as part of a personal wellness program.

Handout 15:2 - EXERCISE GUIDELINES FOR HEALTH-RELATED PHYSICAL FITNESS

	TYPE OF EXERCISE (What Kind of Exercise)	INTENSITY (How Hard)	DURATION (How Long)	FREQUENCY (How Often)
CARDIORESPIRATORY FITNESS	Use large muscle groups Rhythmic Continuous	60% to 90% of Maximum Heart Rate*	20 to 60 Minutes	3 to 5 Days Per Week
BODY COMPOSITION (For Loss of Excess Body Fat)	Use large muscle groups Rhythmic Continuous	60% to 80% of Maximum Heart Rate*	30 to 60 Minutes	5 to 7 Days Per Week
MUSCLE STRENGTH (Gain or maintain Muscle Tissue)	Use large muscle groups Full Range of Movement Against Resistance	70% to 100% of Maximum Voluntary Contraction**	1 to 10 Repetitions 1 to 3 Sets	2 to 3 Days Per Week
MUSCLE ENDURANCE	Use large muscle groups Full Range of Movement Against Resistance	50% to 70% of Maximum Voluntary Contraction**	20 to 50 Repetitions 1 to 3 Sets	2 to 3 Days Per Week
FLEXIBILITY	Static Stretch	Moderate Discomfort	Hold 10 to 30 Seconds Repeat 1 to 3 Times	3 to 7 Days Per Week

*(Estimated Maximum Heart Rate = 220 minus age)

**Maximum Voluntary Contraction = One Repetition Maximum

Developed by: Dr. James Hesson, Professor of Biology and Biokinetics, Black Hills State University

Adapted from American College of Sports Medicine (ACSM) and National Strength and Conditioning Association (NSCA) Guidelines.

ACTIVITY 5 - DIETARY GUIDELINES

Objectives: The purpose of this activity is to give you an opportunity to assess your nutritional habits and compare them to the recommendations in *Dietary Guidelines for Americans 2005*.

Instructions: Explore the *Dietary Guidelines* website at
http://www.healthierus.gov/dietaryguidelines/
Look at the key recommendations and the frequently asked questions, as well as other links that catch your interest. Write a short paper comparing your nutritional behavior to each of the recommendations in the *Dietary Guidelines*. Include the areas you identify as needing the most improvement.

You could add to this assignment by keeping a food diary for several days to increase your awareness of current eating patterns. Include your emotional state or how you are feeling when you eat to help identify patterns of eating related to stress or emotions.

RELATED WEBSITES

Exercise as a Stress Management Modality
A paper on how physical activity can function as a therapeutic modality. Also included are recommendations on the use of physical activity to promote emotional health.
http://www.imt.net/~randolfi/ExerciseStress.html

Dietary Guidelines for Americans 2005
Dietary Guidelines for Americans is published jointly every 5 years by the Department of Health and Human Services (HHS) and the Department of Agriculture (USDA). The *Guidelines* provide authoritative advice for people two years and older about how good dietary habits can promote health and reduce risk for major chronic diseases.
http://www.healthierus.gov/dietaryguidelines/

Stress and Nutrition
Stress may increase your body's need for certain nutrients and weaken your immune system, so you may need an extra healthy diet to stay focused, alert, energetic and to ward off colds and flu. This website gives useful information for doing just that.
http://www.uhs.uga.edu/stress/nutrition.html

Why stress can make you fat
Dr. Pamela Peeke, a former researcher on stress and nutrition at the National Institute of Health, discusses the connection between stress and weight control.
http://www.inq7.net/lif/2003/jun/03/text/lif_21-1-p.htm

Sleep and Stress
Interesting website on the effects of sleep on stress.
http://www.fi.edu/brain/sleep.htm

CHAPTER 16
INTRODUCTION TO RELAXATION

CHAPTER OUTLINE
Use this outline to take notes as you read the chapter in the text and/or as your instructor lectures in class.

I.   INTRODUCTION TO RELAXATION
       A. Despite our best efforts to prevent it, stress happens.
       B. If you are living a typical modern-day life, stress is almost unavoidable.
           1. Therefore, we need tools that we can immediately use to turn the stress response
               off and consequently, avoid the large number of unpleasant health problems
               associated with chronic stress.
       C. Through the rest of the book you will learn effective and powerful ways to reduce stress
           and tension through techniques that are designed to cancel the effects of stress arousal by
           putting your body into a relaxed state.

II.   UNDERSTANDING RELAXATION
       A. There are many good definitions of relaxation
           1. For this text, **relaxation** is the mind/body process of effectively moving from the
               stress response to the relaxation response.
           2. Relaxation is the opposite of the stress response.
       B. Effort is involved to create true relaxation.
           1. Fortunately, the kind of effort involved in stress management is the kind that
               produces pleasant, positive results.
           2. The purpose of relaxation techniques is to directly activate parasympathetic
               nervous system activity.
       C. Relaxation is not the same thing as watching television, reading a good book, or even
           viewing a sunset.
           1. It is also not the same thing as daydreaming or letting the mind wander aimlessly.
               a) It is easy to do these things and they might seem pleasant and enjoyable,
                   but they aren't necessarily designed to activate the relaxation response.
       D. Relaxation techniques work by deliberately canceling the arousal of the nervous system,
           the muscles and the mind.
           1. The relaxed state is the opposite of the stressed state, therefore it is not possible
               to be both stressed and relaxed.
       E. In Part 4 of this book you will discover a wide assortment of relaxation techniques that you
           can immediately include in your busy days to help reduce stress.
       F. As you begin to practice and experiment with them, here are some important points to
           keep in mind:
           1. Not every relaxation technique works the same for everyone.
           2. You should try each method several times.
           3. Regardless of how strange they may appear to you, each has been found to be
               effective.

III.   BENEFITS OF RELAXATION
       A. Relaxation can improve how your body responds to stress by:
           1. Slowing your heart rate, meaning less work for your heart
           2. Reducing blood pressure
           3. Slowing your breathing rate
           4. Reducing the need for oxygen
           5. Increasing blood flow to the major muscles
           6. Lessening muscle tension
       B. After practicing relaxation skills, you may experience the following benefits:
           1. Fewer symptoms of illness, such as headaches, nausea, diarrhea and pain.
           2. Fewer emotional responses such as anger, crying, anxiety, apprehension and

frustration.
3. More energy.
4. Improved concentration.
5. Greater ability to handle problems.
6. More efficiency in daily activities.

C. Many health benefits result from relaxation.
   1. As you learn to relax, you will become more aware of muscle tension and other physical sensations caused by the stress response.
   2. In time, you may even notice your body's reaction before you take mental note of your stress.

IV. **GETTING STARTED**

A. With most of these relaxation methods, there are things you can do to make your experience more pleasant and effective.
   1. Seclude yourself where you will not be interrupted.
   2. Minimize background noises.
   3. Give yourself ten to twenty minutes each day practicing a relaxation activity.
      a) Consider the fact that practicing relaxation exercises is as important to your health and well-being as being physically active or eating a healthy diet.
   4. Practice the relaxation techniques during the times of the day recommended for each one.
      a) Some are more appropriately done in the morning, while others seem to have a more positive effect in the afternoon or right before going to sleep.
   5. Do not be in any hurry to end the relaxation exercise.
      a) If you hurry to finish a relaxation exercise, it will feel much much the same as you feel when you awaken from a deep sleep to a ringing telephone.
         (1) Hurrying to end a relaxation exercise is disruptive and can leave you feeling off balance for the rest of the day.
      b) If you are using the Stress Relief DVD, follow the pace of the guide.
      c) If you are doing it on your own, take several minutes to return to normal waking consciousness.
   6. Turn off the telephone, your cell phone, and any device that might have an alarm.
   7. Approach each exercise without expectations; be playful with them.
      a) The best attitude to have when you do the exercises is one of openness to whatever results you experience.
      b) As you practice, say to yourself, "I will take what I get. If I get nothing, then that is what I get ... and that's okay. If I get some deep rest and relaxation, then that is what I get as well. It's also okay if I feel rejuvenated and energized."
      c) Trying too hard to make them work counteracts the desired effects.
   8. Regardless of how new or unusual any of these exercises might seem to you, they have been found to be effective in turning off the stress response and restoring balance.
      a) If you notice yourself resisting an exercise because it seems too unusual, simply thank that part of your mind for sharing its judgmental thoughts with you and continue in a playful, childlike way.
      b) Don't let the possibly strange nature of the method prevent you from experiencing it fully.
   9. The most important aspect of a relaxation exercise is not what happens during it but how you feel *after completing the exercise.*
      a) Don't judge a relaxation technique based on what happens during it.
         (1) You may not always feel relaxed while you are practicing.
         (2) Your mind may feel like it is moving a million miles a minute or you may be quite physically involved, as is the case when you practice

progressive relaxation.
   b) Relaxation exercises work so that when you are through and into the activities of your day you feel more balanced, alert, relaxed, refreshed and have more energy.

10. Science cannot fully explain why some of these relaxation exercises work so well.
   a) Deep relaxation happens even without full understanding.
      (1) It is not always necessary to understand why the process works to enjoy the positive benefits.

V.   **UNUSUAL SENSATIONS**
   A. Occasionally, individuals experience unusual sensations while practicing relaxation exercises.
      1. Tingling
      2. Warmth
      3. Coolness
      4. Floating
      5. Swirling
      6. Spinning
      7. Heaviness
      8. A pleasant numbness or seeming inability to move a part of the body
      9. More pronounced heartbeat
      10. Distortions in your sense of time (you may perceive time moving extremely fast or slow – usually fast)
      11. Lightheadedness
   B. These sensations typically feel pleasant and are natural responses to the body turning off the stress response and restoring balance to body systems.
      1. They are indications that you are doing the exercises correctly; you have achieved deep relaxation.
      2. When you experience any of these sensations, simply go with them and observe what happens.
         a) Don't resist them.
      3. Whatever happens while you are relaxing, according to the instructions in this book or on the DVD, is entirely appropriate for you.
         a) Allow these sensations to happen freely.
      4. Most of the time you will experience little if anything unusual while you are practicing, but occasionally, you will.
   C. One byproduct of regular practice of relaxation exercises is the possibility that you may not need to take as many medications as you are presently.
      1. Many of the symptoms of stress are alleviated with regular practice.

VI.   **TIME FOR A NAP ... A POWER NAP**
   A. The first relaxation technique, the **Power Nap** combines elements of several relaxation exercises, including deep breathing, mindfulness, and yoga to relax and rejuvenate both body and mind.
      1. The benefits of this relaxation technique, more than just about any other, include an immediate increase in energy, an increase in ability to focus, and a general feeling of rejuvenation.
      2. If the Power Nap is done just prior to falling asleep, it can result in falling asleep quickly and remaining asleep throughout the night for a deeply restful sleep.

VII.   **HOW TO DO THE POWER NAP**
   A. The Power Nap is simple. All that is required is a soft floor, a chair, a couch, or a bed, and some privacy so you will not be interrupted. Figure 16.1 demonstrates the body position for the Power Nap.
      1. These ten easy steps will guide you through the Power Nap.
         a) Follow the directions listed in this section of the chapter.
   B. There are a couple of "best times" during the day to do the Power Nap:

1. Late afternoon after your day's activities and before evening activities.
2. Just before falling asleep.
    a) Complete your normal bedtime routine.
    b) Make the Power Nap the last thing that you do before your head hits the pillow and you close your eyes.
        (1) Once you have finished this relaxation exercise, slip into bed and easily fall asleep.

VIII.   **CONCLUSION**
A. Relaxation is the mind/body process of effectively moving from the stress response to the relaxation response.
    1. Benefits occur when we move from physical and psychological arousal to relaxation.
    2. The purpose of relaxation techniques is to directly activate calming parasympathetic nervous system activity.
B. The Power Nap is a simple yet powerful technique to activate the relaxation response by combining elements of deep breathing, mindfulness, and yoga.
C. Each time you participate in one of the relaxation techniques, think of it as taking a mini-vacation from stress.

LEARNING ACTIVITIES

ACTIVITY 1 - JOURNALING

Objective: The purpose of this activity is to encourage critical thinking and honest personal reflection on topics relating to the chapter content. Explore personal thoughts, feelings, values, and behaviors as you selectively incorporate stress management knowledge and behaviors into your plan for improved health through better stress management.

Instructions: You will find journaling questions in each chapter of your Activities Manual. These questions relate specifically to the chapter content. Moving your thoughts from your mind to the paper is a powerful strategy for relieving stress and for increasing awareness of your thoughts, feelings and behaviors. Your course instructor can provide further guidance on how to complete this activity.

Complete the following journaling questions. Select the questions that have the most relevance for you.

1. Why do you think the Power Nap works to facilitate relaxation and manage stress? List as many reasons as you can come up with to explain why this might work.
2. What appear to be the primary differences between cognitive techniques to prevent the stress response and physical techniques to reduce the stress response? Why do you think there is value in having a variety of strategies that work for you in different situations?
3. After you have tried the Power Nap a couple times, take time to write a detailed reflection on how you feel when you are done. Include body, mind and spirit results.
4. How does the information in this chapter affect you personally? What insights did you have about yourself and the stress that you experience?

ACTIVITY 2 - INTRODUCTION TO RELAXATION

Objectives: The purpose of this activity is to inform you of ways to create the most favorable conditions for relaxation exercises.

Description of Activity: When preparing for and practicing relaxation exercises consider these guidelines:

*   Seclude yourself where you will not be interrupted.
*   Minimize background noises.
*   Give yourself ten to twenty minutes each day practicing a relaxation activity. Consider the fact that practicing relaxation exercises is as important to your health and well-being as being physically active or eating a healthy diet.
*   Practice the relaxation techniques during the times of the day recommended for each one. Some are more appropriately done in the morning, while others seem to have a more positive effect in the afternoon or right before going to sleep.
*   Do not be in any hurry to end the relaxation exercise. This is important. If you hurry to finish a relaxation exercise, it will feel much like the way you feel when you awaken from a deep sleep to a ringing telephone. Hurrying to end a relaxation exercise is disruptive and can leave you feeling off balance for the rest of the day. If you are using the Stress Relief DVD, follow the pace of the guide. If you are doing it on your own, take several minutes to return to normal waking consciousness. Hurrying to finish can spoil all the work that you do resting and restoring your mind and body during a relaxation exercise.
*   Turn off the telephone, your cell phone, and any device that might have an alarm.
*   Approach each exercise without expectations; be playful with them. The best attitude to have when you do the exercises is one of openness to whatever results you experience. As you practice, say to yourself, "I will take what I get. If I get nothing, then that is what I get ... and that's okay. If I get some deep rest and relaxation, then that is what I get as well. It's also okay if I feel rejuvenated and energized." Trying too hard to make them work counteracts the desired effects.

- Regardless of how new or unusual any of these exercises might seem to you, they have been found to be effective in turning off the stress response and restoring balance. If you notice yourself resisting an exercise because it seems too unusual, simply thank that part of your mind for sharing its judgmental thoughts with you and continue in a playful, childlike way. Don't let the possibly strange nature of the method prevent you from experiencing it fully.
- The most important aspect of a relaxation exercise is not what happens during it but how you feel *after completing the exercise.* Don't judge a relaxation technique based on what happens during it. You may not always feel relaxed while you are practicing. Your mind may feel like it is moving a million miles a minute or you may be quite physically involved, as is the case when you practice progressive relaxation. Relaxation exercises work so that when you are through and into the activities of your day you feel more balanced, alert, relaxed, refreshed and have more energy.
- Science cannot fully explain why some of these relaxation exercises work so well. Autogenics and meditation are good examples of this. Science has not yet figured out why the simple repetition of a word produces such deep and profound rest, but deep relaxation happens even without full understanding. The person who goes into the gym to lift weights to make her body stronger may have no idea why her muscles seem to get bigger when she lifts heavy weights for many repetitions. That may not matter to her if what she is interested in is the results. Lifting weights produces the results she is seeking. Similarly, with relaxation exercises, it is not always necessary to understand why the process works to enjoy the positive benefits.

ACTIVITY 3 - RELAXATION EXERCISE - THE POWER NAP

Relaxation Activity: The Power Nap

Objectives: The purpose of this activity is to allow you to practice deep relaxation on your own using the Power Nap

Materials needed:
Stress Relief DVD
Handout 16:1 - DVD Relaxation Exercise - the Power Nap

Instructions:
1. Practice the Power Nap at least twice on your own following the instructions on the DVD. At least once (and preferably more frequently) do it immediately before falling asleep.

2. Assess your experience by following the instructions on Handout 16:1 - DVD Relaxation Exercise - the Power Nap.

Handout 16:1 - DVD Relaxation Exercise
The Power Nap

The DVD homework assignment for this week is the first exercise on the Stress Relief DVD called the "Power Nap"

Practice doing this exercise at least two (2) times according to the instructions on the DVD. One of those times, do it immediately before you get into bed to sleep at night. Make it the very last thing you do before your head hits your pillow.

Do it at times when you will not be disturbed. It lasts approximately 15 minutes.

In a *typed* format, you will respond to the following items:

1. How you felt before the exercise
2. Your experience during the exercise
3. How you felt immediately following the exercise
4. How you felt long after completing the exercise, or how you slept and awakened the following morning

On your typed paper, **thoroughly** respond to each of these items referring to the two times that you did them at home, *and* the time that you did it in class. Describe primarily how you were feeling in relation to your stress levels.

Follow this general outline with your description:

Afternoon:
- Before
- During
- Immediately after
- Long after

Right before bed:
- Before
- How quickly you fell asleep
- How you slept
- How refreshed you felt in the morning
- How this differed from a typical night's sleep

Classroom experience (if applicable):
- Before
- During
- Immediately after
- Long after

RELATED WEBSITES

Coping with Stress: Management and Reduction Techniques
Website that discusses a variety of ways to manage stress
http://www.helpguide.org/mental/stress_management_relief_coping.htm

Relaxation: Calming the Nervous System
Website describes the benefits of regular relaxation for people with chronic conditions.
http://www.tenresolutions.org/2-3.html

Stress Management May Save Lives
Article that suggests the value of stress management for cardiac patients
http://www.law.berkeley.edu/administration/hr/worklife/stress-management.pdf

CHAPTER 17
TAKE A BREATH

CHAPTER OUTLINE
Use this outline to take notes as you read the chapter in the text and/or as your instructor lectures in class.

I.   TAKE A BREATH
     A.   Breath is life!
     B.   Breathing represents an important point of contact between mind and body, since respiration occupies a unique interaction between the voluntary and involuntary nervous systems.
     C.   Shallow and irregular breathing reinforces stress and can have negative physical consequences.
     D.   Deep breathing, however, induces relaxation and promotes circulation.
     E.   In our busy lives, we continually inhibit our natural breathing patterns in many ways, including habitual patterns of emotional stress.
          1.   Conscious relaxation breathing relieves stress, allowing a return to natural, uninhibited breathing.

II. BACKGROUND
     A.   For centuries, breathing exercises have been an integral part of mental, physical, and spiritual development in Asia and India.
     B.   Deep breathing continues to be an essential component of ancient Eastern practices such as yoga and tai chi chuan.
     C.   Breathing techniques are part of a philosophical system that emphasizes balance and wholeness for achieving health.

III. HOW BREATHING WORKS
     A.   The primary purpose of breathing is to supply the body with oxygen and to remove excess carbon dioxide.
          1.   The body's ability to produce energy and to complete the various metabolic processes depends upon sufficient and efficient use of oxygen.
               a)   Oxygen is necessary to help us repair and regenerate our bodies.
          2.   An average human breath contains about 10 sextillion or 10^{22} atoms.
               a)   If any tissues in the body, including the heart and the brain, are deprived of oxygen for more than a few minutes, severe damage can occur.
     B.   There are two basic ways of breathing: one is **abdominal, or diaphragmatic, breathing**; the other is **chest, or thoracic, breathing**.
          1.   Chest breathing is relatively shallow.
               a)   The chest expands and the shoulders rise as the lungs take in air.
               b)   Thoracic or chest breathing is frequently a signal that the fight-or-flight response is activated even to the point of holding the breath or exhaling incompletely.
                    (1) People who have chronic stress tend to breathe either with their chest almost exclusively, or both with their abdomen and chest simultaneously.
          2.   Abdominal breathing is deeper.
               a)   Abdominal diaphragmatic breathing involves inhalations that cause the **diaphragm** to contract and move down, drawing air into the lungs.
                    (1) When air moves down into the lungs at the lower levels, the abdomen tends to distend slightly.
                    (2) On exhalation, the diaphragm relaxes and moves upward and the abdomen moves back in.
               b)   Breathing abdominally helps bring air into the lower lobes of the lungs, resulting in an increase in beneficial oxygenation throughout the various

cells and systems of the body.

      c) We are born as abdominal breathers; it is our natural way of breathing.

IV. BENEFITS OF RELAXATION BREATHING

A. The natural breathing process shows great promise as a coping technique for common anxiety and stress.

    1. Slow, rhythmic breathing can turn an anxious mental state into one of relative tranquility and release the body from many other adverse effects of anxiety.

        a) Adjusting our breathing back to its naturally deep and slow way sends an instant message to the autonomic nervous system that there is no threat and the body can return to homeostasis.

            (1) When the body returns to a more balanced state, turning off the fight or flight response, a balance is created where the body can cure its maladies associated with stress.

            (2) Deep abdominal breathing is not only effective in reducing levels of stress and coping with stressful situations including test anxiety, but also in reducing blood pressure.

    2. A number of studies have been done to show the effectiveness of deep breathing in turning off the stress response and as a result, decreasing the symptoms associated with chronic stress.

B. Nearly every stress management technique that is specifically created to reduce sympathetic nervous activity includes a breathing component.

V. HOW TO DO RELAXATION BREATHING

A. Breathing exercises may be practiced lying down or sitting in a comfortable chair.

B. Practice breathing exercises in a room that is quiet and conducive to relaxation.

C. Breathing exercises are best done with the eyes closed.

D. Any time of the day is an appropriate time to practice breathing relaxation exercises, but they can be particularly beneficial in the afternoon or just before going to sleep.

    1. Relaxing breathing exercises can be especially effective in helping one fall asleep.

    2. Adjusting from chest breathing to deeper abdominal breathing can be done anytime and anywhere.

VI. BREATHING EXERCISES

A. **Simple Diaphragmatic Breathing** can be done by placing one hand on the stomach, approximately over the navel, and the other on the lower part of the sternum just over the heart.

    1. Notice which hand is moving more, the upper or the lower hand, during inhalation and exhalation.

    2. Make the hand over the stomach move out with the inhalation and in with the exhalation, while the top hand remains still.

    3. For added benefit, try repeating "I am" with each inhalation and "relaxed" with each exhalation.

B. **Reduce Respirations Technique** works to reduce your breathing rate to between 10 and 12 breaths per minute and even slower if possible.

    1. Take a deep, slow breath, drawing in through the nose and out through the mouth, which should be closed when inhaling. Inhaling and exhaling should take about six seconds each.

    2. Place one hand over the diaphragm area of the abdomen and continue drawing long, slow, deep breaths using the same method. Aim to reduce breathing to 10-12 breaths per minute.

    3. While breathing deeply through the nose, the hand should move up and down as the chest wall expands and contracts with lung inflation and deflation. Shoulders should remain stationary.

    4. Continue this exercise for several minutes once the desired breathing rate has been achieved.

C. **Restful Breathing** can be done whenever you think of it.
   1. Begin Restful Breathing by focusing directly on your breath as it goes in and comes back out. This may be done with the eyes open or closed. Don't try to change anything about your breathing initially, just tune in to the rhythmic in and out pattern of your breathing. Keep your attention on your breathing.
   2. When your mind wanders and distracting thoughts arise, let them pass, and return your focus to your breath. You may want to place your hands on your abdomen to increase your focus on abdominal breathing.
   3. After a few minutes of attentive breathing, begin to change your breathing pattern by allowing your breath to go down as deep as possible in to the lowest parts of your lungs. When you do this, your abdomen will naturally move outward. Notice your hands, which are resting on your abdomen, moving out as you breathe in. Notice your hands moving back in as you exhale.
   4. To help you maintain your focus on this deep, slow breathing, use the counting method. Start counting at 20 (or whatever number you choose) and count backwards to zero. When you inhale, silently say the number "20." When you exhale, mentally say the word "relax." Inhale again and say the number "19." On the next exhalation, say "relax." Continue down this way until you reach zero.
   5. If you notice your mind starting to wander, and it very likely will, gently bring yourself back to the counting. Your breathing will naturally become more slow and deep as you do this. You can also consciously make your breathing more slow and deep just by focusing on that mode of breathing.

D. **Breath Counting** is similar to restful breathing with slight variations
   1. Simply focus directly on the breath as it comes in and goes back out.
   2. You inhale, and then as you exhale, you say the number "1."
   3. The next inhalation is followed by the exhalation and saying the number "2."
   4. You continue through the number 4 and then repeat again from 1 to 4.

E. **Alternating Nostril Breathing** (also known as balanced breathing) relaxes the mind and body and enhances one's experience of meditation.
   1. The thumb and forefinger are used in this technique to alternate pressing on either side of the nose.
      a) The focus is placed directly on the breath as you alternately exhale and inhale through one nostril, then exhale and inhale through the other nostril.
   2. Beginning with the exhalation, push the thumb against one side of the nose to shut off that nostril as air passes freely through the other.
   3. During the following inhalation, continue to hold the nostril closed.
   4. On the next exhalation, release the thumb and push against the nose with the forefinger on the opposite nostril closing this one off completely.
   5. Inhale while holding the same nostril occluded.
   6. This pattern, switching back and forth from one nostril to the other, can be repeated as long as desired.

F. With **Patterned Breathing**, maintain a complete focus on the breath as it goes in, hold the breath for a short period, follow this with the exhalation, and finish the patterned breath with a final pause before the next breath begins again.
   1. One common pattern is the 1-4-4-1 breathing pattern.
      a) The 1-4-4-1 pattern is modified to the desired length of each segment of the breath.
   2. This rhythm would start with an inhalation to a count of 3, for example.
   3. Next the breath is held to a count of 12.
   4. This is followed by exhaling very slowly to a count of 12.
   5. Before inhaling again, pause to a count of 3.

G. **Full Breathing** involves breathing in first to the abdomen and then slowly filling up the rest of the lungs as you inhale.

1. After holding your breath for a few moments, you exhale by first releasing the air from the tops of the lungs and then slowly move down to the lower parts of the lungs so the abdomen moves back in at the end of the exhalation.

H. **Visualization Breathing** combines Full Breathing with visualization.
   1. As you inhale, visualize the in-breath moving down from your nose to the deepest parts of your lungs.
      a) If it helps to visualize it more clearly, imagine your breath is colored, such as white.
   2. After a full inhale, hold the breath briefly and visualize it becoming energized in the lower parts of your lungs.
   3. As you begin slowly exhaling, visualize this energized air spreading to all parts of your body, bringing with it healing energy and purified oxygen.
   4. On the next inhalation, repeat this process.

I. **Command Breathing** can be done on one's own or with the help of a guide.
   1. Take a deep breath, hold it for a few moments, then at the command of the guide release it completely.
   2. The next time the command breath is taken, focus all distraction, tension, and discomfort into that breath and let it all go with the exhalation.
      a) Let everything flow out with the air leaving the lungs.
   3. Repeat the Command Breathing process about two to four times.
      a) Each time imagine and believe that all distraction is passed out of the body and mind with each exhalation.

J. **Ujjayi Breathing** is commonly used while practicing yoga.
   1. It is an audible breath that has a soothing, rhythmic, oceanic quality.
   2. It is done by contracting the whispering muscles in your throat to create a long, hairline thin breath.
   3. You do not breathe all the way down into your abdomen, but rather into your chest, lungs, and back.
      a) Bring your first or second finger to the soft spot between your collarbones.
      b) With your mouth closed, breathe in through your nose, feeling the gentle retraction of those muscles beneath your finger.
         (1) It should feel as though you are whispering in reverse.
         (2) You are closing the airway a little, so it's kind of like breathing through a straw.
         (3) Imagine the breath as a cleansing wind sweeping right in through that soft spot at the base of your throat.
      c) For the exhalation, put your hand in front of your face as if it's a mirror.
         (1) Gently retract your belly and, with your mouth closed and the muscles in your throat still contracted, exhale through your nose as if you were going to fog up that mirror.
         (2) The exhalation is exaggerated and extended. It is important to keep your mouth closed or you will lose energy on the exhalation.

K. Breathing while stretching targets whole-body tension, diverting attention away from anxiety-related physiological sensations toward feelings of relaxation and calmness.
   1. Mentally scan yourself for tension and rate yourself on a 1-100 scale for anxiety.
   2. Stand or sit in a chair with your back straight.
   3. Raise your arms, parallel to your sides, until they are directly overhead. Clasp your hands together and stretch toward the ceiling.
      a) While raising your hands upward, inhale slowly and deeply though the mouth, with lungs full when the hands reach their apex.
      b) Hold your breath for 3-5 seconds while stretching upward.
   4. Slowly exhale through the nose while lowering hands back to your sides.
   5. Intertwine the fingers of both hands and with palms facing outward push away from the chest, arms parallel to the floor.

a) While pushing away, take a deep breath through the mouth.

b) When arms reach maximum extension, push away from them, stretching the back and arms, holding the breath for 3-5 seconds.

6. Return the arms slowly to their resting position while exhaling slowly through the nose.

7. Repeat this exercise 3-5 times. Rate your body sensations and perceptions of anxiety on a 1-100 scale.

8. Repeat as necessary.

VII. CONCLUSION

A. Conscious breathing is a component of nearly every relaxation technique.

1. Used alone, or in combination with other techniques, the beneficial results are immediately obvious.

B. The main focus in directing attention toward the breath is to consciously return breathing to its natural rhythm of deep, slow, and effortless inhaling and exhaling.

1. As we do this, the stress response automatically turns off just as efficiently as it turns on when we sense any kind of danger or potential pain.

<u>LEARNING ACTIVITIES</u>

ACTIVITY 1 - JOURNALING

Objective: The purpose of this activity is to encourage critical thinking and honest personal reflection on topics relating to the chapter content. Explore personal thoughts, feelings, values, and behaviors as you selectively incorporate stress management knowledge and behaviors into your plan for improved health through better stress management.

Instructions: You will find journaling questions in each chapter of your Activities Manual. These questions relate specifically to the chapter content. Moving your thoughts from your mind to the paper is a powerful strategy for relieving stress and for increasing awareness of your thoughts, feelings and behaviors. Your course instructor can provide further guidance on how to complete this activity.

Complete the following journaling questions. Select the questions that have the most relevance for you.

1. What do you think are the physiological and psychological explanations for the effectiveness of breathing in promoting relaxation?
2. After you have tried several different breathing techniques, discuss the breathing technique that seemed to work the best at helping you feel more relaxed.
3. Prior to your next exam in any class, try one of the breathing techniques to initiate the relaxation response. After doing this, what were your results?
4. How does the information in this chapter affect you personally? What insights did you have about yourself and the stress that you experience?

ACTIVITY 2 - RELAXATION EXERCISE - RESTFUL BREATHING

Objectives: The purpose of this activity is to allow you to practice deep relaxation on your own using the Restful Breathing relaxation exercise

Materials needed:
Stress Relief DVD
Handout 17:1 - DVD Relaxation Exercise - Restful Breathing

Instructions:
1. Practice Restful Breathing at least two times on your own following the instructions on the DVD. At least once (and preferably more frequently) do it immediately before falling asleep.

2. Assess your experience by following the instructions on the worksheet Handout 17:1 - DVD Relaxation Exercise - Restful Breathing.

Handout 17:1 - DVD Relaxation Exercise
Restful Breathing

The DVD homework assignment for this week is the fourth exercise on the Stress Relief DVD called "Restful Breathing."

Practice doing this exercise at least two (2) times according to the instructions on the DVD. One of those times, do it immediately before you fall asleep at night. Make it the very last thing you do before you close your eyes to fall asleep.

Do it at times when you will not be disturbed. It lasts approximately 12 minutes.

In a *typed* format, respond to the following items:

1. How you felt before the exercise
2. Your experience during the exercise
3. How you felt immediately following the exercise
4. How you felt long after completing the exercise, or how you slept and awakened the following morning

On your typed paper, **thoroughly** respond to each of these items referring to the two times that you did them at home, *and* the time that you did it in class. Describe primarily how you were feeling in relation to your stress levels.

Follow this general outline with your description:

Afternoon:
- Before
- During
- Immediately after
- Long after

Right before bed:
- Before
- How quickly you fell asleep
- How you slept
- How refreshed you felt in the morning
- How this differed from a typical night's sleep

Classroom experience (if applicable):
- Before
- During
- Immediately after
- Long after

ACTIVITY 3 – MINI RELAXATION BREAK

Objectives: The purpose of this activity is to give you a quick relaxation break using a relaxing breathing technique.

Instructions: This activity can be done at any time when you are feeling a little bit tense and need to relax.

You can do this any time you are seated. It can be done with eyes open or closed. Simply take a few minutes and practice any of the breathing exercises outlined in chapter 17 of the textbook. Do them very mindfully—if your mind wanders, simply return your thoughts to your breath and the pattern of breathing you have selected to practice.

You don't need to do this for much longer than 5 minutes. Try to sense the length of time that seems appropriate to you.

RELATED WEBSITES

Health Hint: Breathing Exercises
Thorough look at breathing as a way of managing stress.
https://www.amsa.org/healingthehealer/breathing.cfm

Relaxation and Chronic Pain
Along with other ways to relax, this site gives additional methods of breathing to bring about relaxation.
http://www.long-beach.med.va.gov/Our_Services/Patient_Care/cpmpbook/cpmp-9.html

Healing Panic
Authoritative self-help information for people who suffer from panic attacks.
http://hope4ever.hypermart.net/start.html

CHAPTER 18
AUTOGENICS

CHAPTER OUTLINE
Use this outline to take notes as you read the chapter in the text and/or as your instructor lectures in class.

I. **AUTOGENICS**
  A. Story of hypnosis at a high school assembly
II. **THE POWER OF SUGGESTION**
  A. The basis for hypnosis is called **suggestion**.
      1. A suggestion is any statement that the mind believes is true, accurate, or real.
  B. The word autogenic comes from the Greek words autos meaning self, and genos meaning origin.
      1. **Autogenics** is self-directed relaxation using suggestions.
III. **BACKGROUND OF AUTOGENIC TRAINING**
  A. **Autogenic training** is a method of reducing the stress response that originated in Europe in the early 20th century by the brain physiologist Oskar Vogt.
      1. Vogt noticed that as his subjects put themselves into a hypnotic state, they experienced substantial decreases in tension, fatigue, and headaches.
  B. Johannes Schultz, a psychiatrist from Germany, continued with the work of Professor Vogt.
      1. Schultz learned that those who were able to attain deep relaxation through hypnosis reported experiencing two pleasant physical sensations.
        a) One was heaviness, and the other was warmth, primarily in their arms and legs.
  C. Schultz developed a system designed to activate the parasympathetic nervous system using suggestions focused on warmth and heaviness.
      1. The simple suggestion to the mind caused the body to respond physically by increasing blood flow to the extremities and relaxing the muscles.
      2. Schultz found that those practicing this simple method were able to attain deep levels of rest similar to those found in people under hypnosis and meditation.
IV. **HOW AUTOGENICS WORKS**
  A. The pleasant feeling of warmth in the extremities can be explained physiologically as the **vasodilation** (increase in the diameter) of blood vessels in response to parasympathetic nervous system activation.
      1. The parasympathetic nervous system is designed to bring the body to a state of homeostasis, or balance.
      2. Vasodilation occurs when the impending threat has passed and there is no longer a need to run or fight.
      3. The pleasant feeling of heaviness is characteristic of muscles, formerly tensed to run or fight, becoming relaxed.
V. **BENEFITS OF AUTOGENICS**
  A. Studies have demonstrated the effectiveness of autogenic training on a variety of stress related problems and maladies.
      1. Reduction of heart rate, blood pressure, respiratory rate, and tension.
      2. Reduction of anxiety, phobic disorders, and hysteria.
      3. Reduction of headaches including tension headaches and migraine headaches.
      4. Reduction in anxiety toward cancer.
      5. Reduction of insomnia and muscle tension.
      6. Decreased effects of post traumatic stress disorder.
      7. Significant improvement in physical performance and significant decrease in physiological arousal.
      8. Reduction of bladder problems, ulcerative colitis, irritable bowel syndrome, diabetes, thyroid disease, grief, eating disorders, PMS, asthma, circulation

disorders, and peptic ulcers.
9. Reduction of mild-to-moderate essential hypertension.
10. Reduction of coronary heart disease.
11. Reduction of bronchial asthma.
12. Reduction of somatoform pain disorder (unspecified type).
13. Reduction of Raynaud's disease.
14. Reduction of anxiety disorders.
15. Reduction of mild-to-moderate depression.
16. Reduction of functional sleep disorders.

VI. **EXPERIENCING AUTOGENICS**
   A. Several factors are important in order for the practice of autogenic training to be successful.
      1. High motivation and cooperation.
      2. A reasonable degree of self-direction and self-control.
      3. Maintenance of a particular body posture conducive to success, including:
         a) Lying on the floor or on a bed (soft flat surface).
         b) Hands resting comfortably at the sides, palms up, fingers loose and extended.
         c) Feet forming a "V" with the heels not quite touching and the toes pointing outward.
         d) The head and neck comfortably supported.
      4. Reduction of external stimuli - turning off all possible sound making devices including cell phones, telephones, television; reducing the possibility of being interrupted by others.
      5. Focus on internal processes to the exclusion of the external environment - focusing attention fully on what is happening internally.
      6. Present the suggestions in a repetitive and monotonous manner, to avoid excitation and to create an environment conducive to passivity
   B. For autogenics to work as intended, a passive attitude is necessary.
      1. Do not "try" to make anything happen.
      2. There should be no conscious effort to force the feelings of warmth, heaviness, or any of the other sensations that are suggested to the mind.
      3. Contrary to some of the other relaxation techniques which involve more willful mental activity, autogenics requires a passive alertness known as **effortless effort**.
   C. The suggestions used in autogenic training usually follow this sequence:
      1. Focus on heaviness in the arms and legs.
      2. Focus on warmth in the arms and legs.
      3. Focus on warmth and heaviness in the heart area.
      4. Focus on breathing.
      5. Focus on coolness in the forehead.

VII. **A SIMPLE AUTOGENICS SCRIPT**
   A. Refer to chapter 18 for an autogenics relaxation script.

VIII. **CONCLUSION**
   A. Autogenics is self-directed relaxation using suggestion.
      1. Pleasant feelings of warmth and heaviness are experienced due to vasodilatation of blood vessels in response to parasympathetic nervous system activation.
      2. Meta-analysis showed autogenic training to be positively beneficial for a variety of conditions, including mood and quality of life.

<u>LEARNING ACTIVITIES</u>

ACTIVITY 1 - JOURNALING

Objective: The purpose of this activity is to encourage critical thinking and honest personal reflection on topics relating to the chapter content. Explore personal thoughts, feelings, values, and behaviors as you selectively incorporate stress management knowledge and behaviors into your plan for improved health through better stress management.

Instructions: You will find journaling questions in each chapter of your Activities Manual. These questions relate specifically to the chapter content. Moving your thoughts from your mind to the paper is a powerful strategy for relieving stress and for increasing awareness of your thoughts, feelings and behaviors. Your course instructor can provide further guidance on how to complete this activity.

Complete the following journaling questions. Select the questions that have the most relevance for you.

1. Many people find a significant decrease in pulse rate after participating in autogenics. When you try autogenics, do you experience a similar drop in resting heart rate? Why do you think this happens?
2. What do you think about the idea of effortless effort? What does this means to you and how does it relate to your experience with autogenics?
3. How does the information in this chapter affect you personally? What insights did you have about yourself and the stress that you experience?

ACTIVITY 2 - RELAXATION EXERCISE - AUTOGENICS

Objectives: The purpose of this activity is to allow you to practice deep relaxation on your own using the Autogenics relaxation exercise.

Materials needed:
Stress Relief DVD
Handout 18:1 - DVD Relaxation Exercise - Autogenics

Instructions:
1. Practice Autogenics at least two times on your own following the instructions on the DVD. At least once (and preferably more frequently) do it immediately before falling asleep.

2. Assess your experience using Handout 18:1 - DVD Relaxation Exercise - Autogenics.

Handout 18:1 - DVD Relaxation Exercise
Autogenics

The DVD homework assignment for this week is the sixth exercise on the Stress Relief DVD called "Autogenics."

Practice doing this exercise at least two (2) times according to the instructions on the DVD. One of those times, do it immediately before you fall asleep at night. Make it the very last thing you do before you close your eyes to fall asleep.

Do it at times when you will not be disturbed. It lasts approximately 18 minutes.

In a *typed* format, respond to the following items:

1. How you felt before the exercise
2. Your experience during the exercise
3. How you felt immediately following the exercise
4. How you felt long after completing the exercise, or how you slept and awakened the following morning

On your typed paper, **thoroughly** respond to each of these items referring to the two times that you did them at home, *and* the time that you did it in class. Describe primarily how you were feeling in relation to your stress levels.

Follow this general outline with your description:

Afternoon:
- Before
- During
- Immediately after
- Long after

Right before bed:
- Before
- How quickly you fell asleep
- How you slept
- How refreshed you felt in the morning
- How this differed from a typical night's sleep

Classroom experience (if applicable):
- Before
- During
- Immediately after
- Long after

<u>**RELATED WEBSITES**</u>

What is Autogenic Training?
Website devoted to information about Autogenics
http://www.autogenics.net/

Autogenics Therapy for Dynamic Relaxation and Stress Relief!
Thorough overview of Autogenic Training
http://www.higher-self-improvement-pursuits.com/autogenics.html

Internet Health Library: Autogenics
Website looks at research showing the effectiveness of autogenics on various maladies.
http://www.internethealthlibrary.com/Therapies/autogenics.htm

CHAPTER 19
PROGRESSIVE RELAXATION

CHAPTER OUTLINE
Use this outline to take notes as you read the chapter in the text and/or as your instructor lectures in class.

I. PROGRESSIVE RELAXATION
    A. Muscle tension may be the most common and annoying symptom of stress.
        1. Stiff neck, tension headache, tight shoulders, grinding teeth, low back pain.
        2. Muscles respond directly to thoughts of perceived danger by tensing in preparation for action.
    B. **Progressive muscle relaxation** (PMR), also known as **progressive neuromuscular relaxation**, is specifically designed to reduce muscle tension.

II. BACKGROUND
    A. While working with patients who suffered from a variety of maladies, Edmund Jacobson noticed one common characteristic in nearly all of his patients: muscle tension.
        1. He found the severity of many disorders could be diminished with reduction or relief of muscle tension.
            a) He found that as his patients were asked to consciously flex these tensed up areas, and then consciously relieve that tension, the contracting muscles would become relaxed.
    B. While Jacobson's original technique has evolved and various adaptations exist, progressive relaxation is one of the most commonly used forms of relaxation therapy in western society today.

III. HOW PMR WORKS
    A. To understand how progressive relaxation works as an effective form of relaxation, it is useful to understand how muscles work.
        1. Skeletal muscles are involved in several physiological functions including generating force (strength and speed), generating heat, maintaining posture and assisting in the breathing process.
        2. A muscle fiber contracts when it receives a nerve impulse from the central nervous system (brain and spinal cord).
            a) After contracting a muscle fiber relaxes until it receives another nerve impulse.
        3. When a **motor unit** gets a message from the nervous system, there is a release of bursts of energy in each of the muscle fibers.
            a) When this occurs, tiny filaments, which are the smallest parts of the muscle, pull on each other and cause a **muscle contraction** or shortening of the muscle fibers.
        4. The **all-or-none principle** of muscle contraction says that a muscle fiber contracts completely or not at all.
            a) Skeletal muscles are naturally in a state of non-contraction, or relaxation.
                (1) When a nervous system signal reaches a muscle motor unit anywhere in the body, all the muscle fibers in this motor unit contract completely.
                (2) When the nerve impulse stops, the contraction stops and the muscle fiber relaxes.

IV. MUSCLES AND RELAXATION
    A. Many muscles in the body remain in a chronically contracted state because they are continuously receiving the message from the nervous system that they should be contracting in preparation for fight or flight.
        1. They don't receive the signal from the nervous system that the threat has passed and it is safe to relax.

2. The modern dilemma is that because our threats do not immediately come to an end, such as daily work pressures, school requirements, or ongoing battles with a partner (all of which are false emergencies), the fight-or-flight response stays activated and therefore, muscle contraction is continuous.

B. Progressive muscle relaxation is designed to initiate parasympathetic nervous system activity in a consciously directed way by first tensing a group of muscles and then consciously releasing the tension in that muscle group.

1. It is called progressive muscle relaxation because one moves progressively through the major areas of the body.

2. Many variations of the original PMR technique exist today, but all have in common the objective of teaching a person to relax the muscles at will by first developing a conscious awareness of what it feels like to be tense and then what it feels like to be relaxed.

V. BENEFITS OF PROGRESSIVE RELAXATION

A. Progressive Relaxation has shown to be beneficial in alleviating or decreasing the following stress-related conditions:

1. Insomnia
2. Post-traumatic stress disorder
3. High heart rate
4. High anxiety levels
5. High levels of perceived stress
6. High levels of salivary cortisol
7. High anxiety
8. Headaches
9. Depression
10. Aversion to chemotherapy
11. Low back pain
12. Hypertension

VI. HOW TO DO PROGRESSIVE MUSCLE RELAXATION

A. **Active progressive relaxation** is done by first tightly tensing up a group of muscles in some part of the body.

1. Once sufficiently contracted, you hold them in this state of near maximal tension for 5 to10 seconds.

B. This is followed by an immediate release of those flexed muscles for fifteen to thirty seconds.

1. During this relaxation phase, consciously relax the muscles even more completely so you are as relaxed as possible.

C. Focus on and notice the difference between tension and relaxation.

D. By tensing your muscles first, you will find that you are able to relax your muscles more than if you tried to relax your muscles directly.

1. Awareness is placed on the sensation of relaxation, resulting from the release of the tension and how this feeling differs from maintained muscular tension.

E. Progressively move through the body, such as the arms, the face, the torso, and the shoulders, tensing and releasing each muscle group as you go.

1. Included on the DVD that accompanies this text is a relaxation exercise titled Progressive Relaxation for you to receive guided practice for this type of relaxation exercise.

F. **Incremental muscle relaxation** changes the process slightly

1. Working through each group of muscles, first tense the muscles maximally to what feels like 100% contraction.

2. After five to ten seconds of contracting maximally, relax that muscle group completely for fifteen to thirty seconds.

3. Make a second contraction of the same muscles this time contracting to what feels like about 50% of maximal contraction.

4. After five to ten seconds of holding this contraction, relax the muscles completely for fifteen to thirty seconds.
5. Create a third contraction of the same muscles but this time flex the muscles at no more than 10% of maximal contraction.
    a) You are barely creating any tension at this point.
6. Hold this for five to ten seconds and then relax the muscles completely for fifteen to thirty seconds.
7. Progress to the next set of muscles and follow the same procedure.

G. A third version of PMR is called **passive progressive relaxation**.
1. It is also known as the **body scan**.
2. This method does not involve active contraction of muscles, but rather a passive scanning of the body.
    a) Attention is placed on a specific area of the body and you simply tune in to what is happening in that part of the body, and then progress to another area of the body.
    b) Remain as passive and non-judgmental as possible, while at the same time, maintaining a detached process of careful observation of body parts, both deep inside and on the surface.
3. You should also become very aware of thoughts which may spontaneously arise while focusing on a specific area of the body.
    a) As thoughts come to the surface, they are noted, but not added to, nor are judgments made about those thoughts.
4. Passive progressive relaxation is a form of meditation.
    a) It is an internal focus similar to methods of meditation described elsewhere in the text.
5. Included on the DVD that accompanies this text is a relaxation exercise titled Flowing Comfort for you to receive guided practice for this type of passive progressive relaxation.

VII. CONCLUSION

A. Many muscles in the body remain in a chronically contracted state when they are continuously receiving the message from the nervous system that they should be contracting in order to fight or run.
1. These muscles do not receive the signal from the nervous system that the threat has passed and it is safe to relax.
2. Active progressive muscle relaxation is a relaxation technique that reduces muscle tension and induces relaxation through first deliberately tensing muscles, and then deliberately relaxing muscles.

B. Passive progressive relaxation is a more passive method of progressing through the various parts of the body using a technique called the body scan.
1. This method does not involve active contraction of muscles, but rather a passive scanning of the body.
2. Through detached awareness and observation individuals discover their bodies in a non-judgmental way and begin to find some relief from their stress-related symptoms.

LEARNING ACTIVITIES

ACTIVITY 1 - JOURNALING

Objective: The purpose of this activity is to encourage critical thinking and honest personal reflection on topics relating to the chapter content. Explore personal thoughts, feelings, values, and behaviors as you selectively incorporate stress management knowledge and behaviors into your plan for improved health through better stress management.

Instructions: You will find journaling questions in each chapter of your Activities Manual. These questions relate specifically to the chapter content. Moving your thoughts from your mind to the paper is a powerful strategy for relieving stress and for increasing awareness of your thoughts, feelings and behaviors. Your course instructor can provide further guidance on how to complete this activity.

Complete the following journaling questions. Select the questions that have the most relevance for you.

1. Consciously contract the muscles of your fist, forearm, and bicep as tightly as you can for about thirty seconds. Hold the contraction as strongly as possible. Now release the muscles in your arm and tune in to the difference that you feel between contraction and relaxation. Notice how tired your arm became and the pain that you felt with this short intense contraction. Consider other muscles around your body that are constantly tensing like your shoulders and back. Based on this understanding and the information in this chapter, how do you think chronic stress contributes to muscle fatigue and pain?
2. The passive progressive relaxation exercise in the chapter contains many of the components treated earlier in the book - especially mindfulness (chapter 7) and simple observation as an effective way of responding (chapter 6). Explain why you think non-judgmental attention toward part of the body might have a relaxing effect on that part of the body.
3. How does the information in this chapter affect you personally? What insights did you have about yourself and the stress that you experience?

ACTIVITY 2 - RELAXATION EXERCISE - PROGRESSIVE RELAXATION

Objectives: The purpose of this activity is to allow you to practice deep relaxation on your own using the Progressive Relaxation exercise

Materials needed:
Stress Relief DVD
Handout 19:1 - DVD Relaxation Exercise - Progressive Relaxation

Instructions:
1. Practice Progressive Relaxation at least two times on your own following the instructions on the DVD. At least once (and preferably more frequently) do it immediately before falling asleep.

2. Assess your experience using Handout 19:1 - DVD Relaxation Exercise - Progressive Relaxation.

Handout 19:1 - DVD Relaxation Exercise
Progressive Relaxation

The DVD homework assignment for this week is the eighth exercise on the Stress Relief DVD called "Progressive Relaxation."

Practice doing this exercise at least two (2) times according to the instructions on the DVD. One of those times, do it immediately before you fall asleep at night. Make it the very last thing you do before you close your eyes to fall asleep.

Do it at times when you will not be disturbed. It lasts approximately 16 minutes.

In a *typed* format, respond to the following items:

1. How you felt before the exercise
2. Your experience during the exercise
3. How you felt immediately following the exercise
4. How you felt long after completing the exercise, or how you slept and awakened the following morning

On your typed paper, **thoroughly** respond to each of these items referring to the two times that you did them at home, *and* the time that you did it in class. Describe primarily how you were feeling in relation to your stress levels.

Follow this general outline with your description:

Afternoon:
- Before
- During
- Immediately after
- Long after

Right before bed:
- Before
- How quickly you fell asleep
- How you slept
- How refreshed you felt in the morning
- How this differed from a typical night's sleep

Classroom experience:
- Before
- During
- Immediately after
- Long after

ACTIVITY 3 - MINI PROGRESSIVE RELAXATION

Objectives: The purpose of this activity is to help you experience the positive benefits of progressive relaxation anytime, anywhere.

Instructions: In any situation in which you find yourself feeling tension, especially muscle tension, take a moment to practice progressive relaxation on your own.

As you inhale, tighten or contract a specific set of muscles in the body to a level of near maximum tension. Then allow the muscles to relax by slowly exhaling as you let the tension release in that part of your body. Repeat this tension and release in the following areas of your body:

Hands and arms - make a tight fist and tighten the muscles through the upper and lower arms.
Face – tighten your eyes as if you were in a sandstorm, tighten your jaw muscles.
Shoulders – push your shoulders up toward your ears as high as possible.
Chest and stomach - tighten the muscles in your chest and stomach.
Upper legs and buttocks - tighten all of these muscle.
Feet – push your toes up as high as possible keeping your heels on the ground.

RELATED WEBSITES

Progressive Relaxation
Self-Administered Progressive Relaxation
http://www.guidetopsychology.com/pmr.htm

Simple Progressive Relaxation Practice
A quick description of how to practice progressive relaxation
http://www.viha.ca/atc/pdf/relaxation_techique.pdf#search='practicing%20progressive%20relaxation'

Body Scan Meditation (BSM)
Discussion of Body Scan Meditation and several types of meditation.
http://www.healthandhealingny.org/complement/meditation.html

CHAPTER 20
GUIDED IMAGERY - USE YOUR IMAGINATION

<u>CHAPTER OUTLINE</u>
Use this outline to take notes as you read the chapter in the text and/or as your instructor lectures in class.

I. **GUIDED IMAGERY - USING YOUR IMAGINATION**
   A. There is no *real* difference between an imagined event and an event that you perceive in your physical experience as far as how your mind interprets its meaning.
      1. If you can imagine yourself relaxing on a beautiful tropical beach in Bora Bora, your body will react as if you are actually there.
      2. On the other hand, you can actually be on a beautiful beach in Bora Bora and if your mind is imagining all you have to do when you get home, your body will react by activating the stress response.
   B. Guided imagery and visualization can direct the imagination in a way that will subdue the sympathetic nervous system and elicit the relaxation response.

II. **BACKGROUND**
   A. Many have discussed the power of the imagination
      1. Einstein said, "Imagination is more important than knowledge."
      2. Jack Nicklaus said, "I never hit a shot, even in practice without this color movie. First I 'see' the ball where I want it to finish, nice and white and sitting up high on the bright green grass. Then the scene quickly changes and I 'see' the ball going there: its path, trajectory, and shape, even its behavior on landing. Then there's a sort of fade-out, and the next scene shows me making the kind of swing that will turn the previous images into reality.
      3. Stephen Covey said, "All things are created twice."
   B. Every voluntary behavior is preceded by an image of what will occur.
      1. The imagined event is as real to the mind as the event that is actually happening in our physical experience.
      2. Whether it is eating a lemon, improving our golf game, or learning to relax, what we first experience in our mind affects our physical experience.

III. **THE MIND AND HOW IT WORKS**
   A. Understanding the theory behind how hypnosis works and the connection between hypnosis and the conscious and subconscious mind will help you understand how relaxation techniques like guided imagery work and why they are so effective for stress reduction.
      1. **Hypnosis** is an altered state of consciousness characterized by extreme suggestibility, relaxation and heightened imagination.
         a) Hypnosis creates a state of deep relaxation and quiets the mind.
         b) Under hypnosis, you can concentrate intensely on a specific thought, memory, feeling or sensation while blocking out distractions.
         c) You are more open than usual to suggestions, and this can be used to improve your health and well-being.
      2. The predominant school of thought on hypnosis is that it is a way to access a person's subconscious mind.
         a) Normally, you are only aware of the thought processes in your conscious mind.
         b) Scientists think that the deep relaxation and focusing exercises of hypnotism work to calm and subdue the conscious mind so that it takes a less active role in your thinking process.
      3. The mind can be broken into two parts - the conscious and the subconscious mind and can be likened to the engineer and the stoker of a coal-powered steam engine train.

a) The conscious mind (engineer) understands such things as right or wrong, good and bad, yes and no and so on, and makes decisions accordingly. This is the choice making part of our mind.

b) The subconscious mind is like the person in the back of the engine who is shoveling coal into the fire - the stoker.

(1) He receives directions from the engineer and does exactly as he is told. (See Figure 20.1)

c) Whatever the conscious mind focuses on, believes, thinks, and directs is what the subconscious mind responds to; it follows through without question.

d) It is the conscious mind that also has doubts, fears, reservations, and considerations about what it feels can or can't be done.

(1) The subconscious mind simply does as it is told.

4. When a person is hypnotized she goes into an altered state of consciousness where the conscious mind, which is more critical and more analytical, is moved off to the side for a little while and the person doing the suggesting talks directly to the subconscious mind. (See Figure 20.2)

a) When the subconscious mind is spoken to directly, without the filtering of the conscious mind, the subconscious simply does as it is told.

(1) It doesn't know limitations, so it does whatever it is told to do.

5. Imagery can be considered to be a form of self-induced hypnosis.

IV. IMAGERY AND VISUALIZATION

A. **Imagery** is a flow of thoughts that includes sensory qualities from one or more of the senses.

B. **Visualization** relates more specifically to using the imagination to picture or see a place or thing.

C. Imagery is a broader term. The more clearly you can imagine the scene and the more senses you involve, the more real it becomes to your mind.

V. USES OF IMAGERY

A. There are several different uses of mental imagery, including the following:

1. Improve performance skills.
2. Improve confidence and positive thinking.
3. Tactical rehearsal and problem solving.
4. Performance review and analysis.
5. Control arousal and anxiety.

VI. RELAXATION GUIDED IMAGERY - WHAT IS IT?

A. **Relaxation guided imagery** is the technique used to connect with the subconscious mind to activate the relaxation response. Guided imagery implies using the imagination in a directed way toward a specific image, scene, or sensation.

1. By imagining a relaxing scene, for example, your mind and body respond as if you were actually in this relaxing spot.

2. This relaxing imagery decreases the arousal of the stimulating, or sympathetic, branch of the autonomic nervous system, which helps reduce anxiety and perception of pain.

B. Guided imagery has been successfully used in these situations or conditions:

1. Athletes, performers, business people, inventors have used guided imagery to help them perform and create.

2. Treating many stress-related symptoms, including headaches, muscle spasms, chronic pain, and general or situation-specific anxiety, asthma, cancer, HIV, migraine headaches, hypertension, and post-surgical healing, and many other stress maladies.

VII. GUIDED IMAGERY AS A TECHNIQUE FOR RELAXATION

    A. The following are some tips for helping make guided imagery an effective way to relax.

        1. Like other methods of relaxation, an appropriate environment is important.

            a) It should be done in a place where you won't be disturbed and where the lights can be turned down.

        2. Some common and very simple images that can help you turn off the stress response include going for a walk along the beach with gentle ocean waves caressing your legs and feet, walking peacefully through a forest, being in the mountains, by a still lake, or sitting by a running river.

        3. You can picture yourself drifting slowly down a lazy stream, sitting atop a silent peak overlooking a majestic view, or resting in the stillness of a quiet field.

            a) There seems to be something very relaxing about seeing ourselves in nature.

        4. You can experiment until you find the most peaceful, relaxing place that you can possibly imagine.

        5. While some people will clearly see a relaxing setting when using R.G.I., for others it will be more illusive and more like a general impression of relaxation.

            a) Some people say they see very clear, sharp images when they close their eyes and imagine something.

            b) Others feel that they don't really 'see' anything, they just sort of 'think about' it or imagine that they are looking at it, or become aware of a feeling impression.

            c) Either way is perfectly fine.

        6. To enhance your experience of relaxation even more, increase the amount of sensory information that you put into your imagination.

            a) By fully and clearly using your senses to imagine scenes that are pleasant and relaxing, you quickly bring feelings of deep relaxation into your mind and body.

        7. Guided imagery is commonly done by having someone read a script or by using a recording that directs your imagination through a relaxing situation or scene.

            a) You may want to simply use your imagination freely on your own to create the scene.

        8. There are some guidelines to ensure a good experience with guided imagery:

            a) Think in terms of the unlimited - there are no limits, no barriers in your imagination. If you want to fly in your imagination, you are free to fly. If you can imagine it... anything is possible.

            b) Release all thoughts of what others might think. There are no "others" in your imagination so don't be shy. Act boldly and freely.

            c) Include relaxing music in the background, such as classical or new age music without lyrics.

            d) Be playful. Don't be too serious when you are working in your imagination.

                (1) The harder you "try," the harder it will be to "view" your imagery well.

        9. A typical script of a guided imagery is found in this part of the chapter.

        10. Included on the DVD that accompanies this text are three relaxation guided imagery exercises for you to receive guided practice.

            a) Guided Imagery - Mountain Lake

            b) Guided Imagery - Inner Wisdom

            c) Guided Imagery - Floating Through Colors.

VIII.   CONCLUSION
A. Guided imagery works in a manner similar to hypnosis to connect directly with the subconscious mind in such a way that your body responds directly to what you are imagining.
   1. Relaxation guided imagery is a technique that you can use to calm your body and mind by suppressing the sympathetic nervous system and creating homeostasis.
   2. If you can imagine yourself relaxing on the beach in Hawaii with a refreshing breeze blowing in from the ocean, you can activate the relaxation response just as if you actually were on the beach relaxing.
B. Remember that it can work both ways; if you actually are on the beach in Hawaii and your mind is imagining all the problems and work you left at home, your body will respond as if you are home dealing with the stresses, and the stress response will be activated.
C. Maybe you can't take a trip to Hawaii, but you can take 20 minutes to imagine you are there. Your body and mind will appreciate the break.

LEARNING ACTIVITIES

ACTIVITY 1 - JOURNALING

Objective: The purpose of this activity is to encourage critical thinking and honest personal reflection on topics relating to the chapter content. Explore personal thoughts, feelings, values, and behaviors as you selectively incorporate stress management knowledge and behaviors into your plan for improved health through better stress management.

Instructions: You will find journaling questions in each chapter of your Activities Manual. These questions relate specifically to the chapter content. Moving your thoughts from your mind to the paper is a powerful strategy for relieving stress and for increasing awareness of your thoughts, feelings and behaviors. Your course instructor can provide further guidance on how to complete this activity.

Complete the following journaling questions. Select the questions that have the most relevance for you.

1. Create an imagery relaxation scenario for yourself. Write it down. Include all your senses in your scenario. Describe as completely as possible the imagery that produces relaxation for you. Reflect on why this is such relaxing imagery for you.
2. Imagery has been described as the doorway to conscious and subconscious reality. Discuss what you think this statement means and how it relates to relaxation.
3. Do a web search on hypnotism. After reading from several sources, explain in your own words how hypnotism might work and how this understanding relates to stress management.
4. Albert Einstein said, "Imagination is more important than knowledge." What do you think he meant by this?
5. What do you think Stephen Covey meant when he said, "All things are created twice?"
6. What do you think the researchers at MIT meant when they suggested that there is no real difference between an imagined event and an event that you perceive in your physical experience as far as how your mind translates its meaning?
7. How have you used imagery to help you accomplish something?
8. After reading through the chapter, explain why you think guided imagery works to bring about relaxation.
9. How does the information in this chapter affect you personally? What insights did you have about yourself and the stress that you experience?

ACTIVITY 2 - RELAXATION EXERCISE - GUIDED IMAGERY
MOUNTAIN LAKE

Objectives: The purpose of this activity is to allow you to practice deep relaxation on your own using the Guided Imagery - Mountain Lake relaxation exercise.

Materials needed:
Stress Relief DVD
Handout 20:1 - DVD Relaxation Exercise - Guided Imagery - Mountain Lake

Instructions:
1. Practice Guided Imagery - Mountain Lake at least two times on your own according to the instructions on the DVD. This exercise is probably best done sitting in a comfortable position rather than lying down. It is not one that is used to help you fall asleep so much as it is used to deeply relax you while remaining conscious.

2. Assess your experience of this exercise using Handout 20:1 - DVD Relaxation Exercise - Guided Imagery - Mountain Lake.

Handout 20:1 - DVD Relaxation Exercise
Guided Imagery – Mountain Lake

The DVD homework assignment for this week is the third exercise on the Stress Relief DVD called "Guided Imagery – Mountain Lake."

Practice doing this exercise at least two (2) times according to the instructions on the DVD. Resist the urge to fall asleep, so ***don't*** do it just before you go to bed.

Do it at times when you will not be disturbed. It lasts approximately 14 minutes.

In a *typed* format, respond to the following items:

1. How you felt before the exercise
2. Your experience during the exercise
3. How you felt immediately following the exercise
4. How you felt long after completing the exercise

On your typed paper, ***thoroughly*** respond to each of these items referring to the two times that you did them at home, *and* the time that you did it in class. Describe primarily how you were feeling in relation to your stress levels.

Follow this general outline with your description:

Daytime (first time):
- Before
- During
- Immediately after
- Long after

Daytime (second time):
- Before
- During
- Immediately after
- Long after

Classroom experience (if applicable):
- Before
- During
- Immediately after
- Long after

ACTIVITY 3 – RELAXATION EXERCISE – GUIDED IMAGERY
FLOATING THROUGH COLORS

Homework Activity: Relaxation Exercise – Guided Imagery - Floating through Colors

Objectives: The purpose of this activity is to allow you to practice deep relaxation on your own using the Guided Imagery - Floating through Colors relaxation exercise.

Materials needed:
Stress Relief DVD
Handout 20:2 DVD Relaxation Exercise – Guided Imagery - Floating through Colors

Instructions:
1. Practice Guided Imagery - Floating through Colors at least two times on your own according to the instructions on the DVD. This exercise is probably best done sitting in a comfortable position rather than lying down. It is not one that is used to help you fall asleep so much as it is used to deeply relax you while remaining conscious.

2. Assess your experience of this exercise using Handout 20:2 DVD Relaxation Exercise - Guided Imagery - Floating through Colors.

Handout 20:2 - DVD Relaxation Exercise
Guided Imagery - Floating through Colors

The DVD homework assignment for this week is the seventh exercise on the Stress Relief DVD called "Guided Imagery - Floating through Colors."

Practice doing this exercise at least two (2) times according to the instructions on the DVD.

Do it at times when you will not be disturbed. It lasts approximately 15 minutes.

In a *typed* format, respond to the following items:

5. How you felt before the exercise
6. Your experience during the exercise
7. How you felt immediately following the exercise
8. How you felt long after completing the exercise

On your typed paper, **thoroughly** respond to each of these items referring to the two times that you did them at home, *and* the time that you did it in class. Describe primarily how you were feeling in relation to your stress levels.

Follow this general outline with your description:

Daytime (first time):
- Before
- During
- Immediately after
- Long after

Daytime (second time):
- Before
- During
- Immediately after
- Long after

Classroom experience (if applicable):
- Before
- During
- Immediately after
- Long after

RELATED WEBSITES

Guided Imagery or Visualization
Good overview of imagery and visualization for stress management and other purposes.
http://holisticonline.com/guided-imagery.htm

Visualization in Sport
Imagery can improve performance
http://sportsmedicine.about.com/cs/sport_psych/a/aa091700a.htm

HealthJourneys: Resources for Mind, Body and Spirit
Try the Audio Spa!
http://www.healthjourneys.com/

CHAPTER 21
MEDITATION

CHAPTER OUTLINE
Use this outline to take notes as you read the chapter in the text and/or as your instructor lectures in class.

I.   MEDITATION: IT'S NOT WHAT YOU *THINK*
     A. Meditation has blossomed into numerous forms practiced by many cultures throughout the centuries.
         1. Many people around the world incorporate some variation of this powerful relaxation technique into their daily routine.
         2. This ancient spiritual practice is finding new uses as both a stress management technique and in the treatment of mental and physical disorders.
II. MEDITATION: WHAT IS IT?
     A. **Meditation** is the process of systematically allowing the mind to focus gently on a single item.
         1. In the process, the mind tends to think more clearly as the mental chatter slows down.
         2. When you clear the clutter from your mind, your mind and body naturally settle to a state of balance, or homeostasis.
         3. The calming mental exercises of meditation are a proven antidote to stress and tension.
     B. Nearly all types of meditation have some characteristics in common:
         1. A quiet environment where you will not be disturbed.
         2. A comfortable, relaxed position, usually sitting.
         3. A point of mental focus.
     C. Meditation may simply mean prayer or contemplation while focusing your mind on a single thought or idea, on an object such as a flower, on a simple shape, on a sound, or on an image.
         1. People have been known to meditate with eyes wide open, while continuously looking at and focusing on the flame of a candle or at one particular point on a wall or ceiling.
     D. Meditation is a powerful and effective means for preventing and reducing stress and the disorders that are associated with chronic stress.
III. WHAT MEDITATION IS NOT
     A. Meditation is not a determined attempt at trying to empty your mind.
         1. Follow the example in chapter 21 of deliberately trying to make the mind go blank.
             a) For most people, this simply is not possible.
             b) Nor is it the goal of meditation.
IV. MEDITATION PUT INTO PRACTICE
     A. Meditation does not take years of practice, nor does it involve venturing off to some spiritually enlightened sage who lives in the Himalayas.
         1. It also does not involve forceful attempts to still the mind.
     B. **Simple meditation** is a technique that combines the following four factors:
         1. A mental device (constant and repetitive focus of attention).
             a) One of the most common mental devices that allows this to happen is called a **mantra** which is simply a repeated word, a sound, or a phrase.
         2. A passive attitude
             a) There should be as little effort as possible when you meditate.
                 (1) Working at meditation does not work.
                 (2) Do not try to make anything happen.
             b) When you meditate, you should have only one intention: the simple act of

repeating the mantra with as little effort exerted as possible.

    (1) Do not try to do anything else or try to make anything else happen.

3. A comfortable position

    a) Meditation begins in a comfortable seated position.

    b) You may choose to sit on the floor, in a chair with a straight back or in a recliner chair, in the **lotus position**, or any other seated position that is comfortable to you.

    c) Try to sit up comfortably straight.

4. A quiet environment

    a) It is beneficial to find a place where you will not be disturbed.

    b) Go into a closet and set your chair there, or go to a room where you know that the phone will not ring and no one will interrupt you.

5. These are the ideal conditions, but with practice, people have been known to practice this type of meditation virtually anywhere, including in airports, cars, boring classes, or at the tops of mountains.

    a) Other environmental noises should not be considered a hindrance to meditation but should be treated the same as your internal thoughts.

6. It is important that you end your meditation correctly to achieve the greatest benefit.

    a) You DO NOT want to come out of meditation quickly.

        (1) If you do, you will feel the same way you do when you are awakened abruptly from a dream.

        (2) You end meditation by returning very slowly to normal consciousness.

        (3) You give yourself two or three full minutes of waking up similar to when you wake up without an alarm on a morning when you are not in any hurry to get up.

        (4) This may sound trivial but it is important.

C. **Breathing meditation** focuses primarily on the breathing, rather than a mantra.

1. The mind is trying neither to forcibly think a certain way nor inhibit thoughts from coming and going.

2. There is simply a calm and passive mental return to focusing on the in-and-out movement of the breath.

3. Most meditation treats rambling thoughts very gently and forgivingly.

4. If thoughts ramble and stray from the intended focus point, there is no criticizing or belittling oneself for not meditating correctly.

    a) The goal is to return and continue putting our attention on our breath.

V. TYPES OF MEDITATION

A. Contemplation

1. In contemplation, the goal is to simply look at the object.

2. There is no attempt to judge the object, or to try to analyze or understand the object. You simply place your attention on it and observe it passively.

B. Breath Counting

1. Breath counting meditation is done by closing your eyes, putting your attention on your breath, and breathing normally.

    a) You inhale, and then when you exhale, you say the number "1."

    b) The next inhale is followed by the exhale and saying the number "2."

    c) You continue through the number 4 and then repeat again from 1 to 4.

    d) You might also include the silently spoken word "and" with each inhale.

        (1) As you inhale, you say the word "and" followed by exhaling to the number.

C. **Thought Watching**
   1. You practice thought watching by picturing yourself sitting peacefully at the bottom of a clear lake.
   2. You begin with the understanding that large bubbles tend to rise from the bottom of the lake to the top in an easy and effortless fashion.
   3. With this idea, tune your attention to your thoughts as they pass into your mind.
   4. As a thought comes in, you picture the thought as a bubble rising slowly and easily to the surface above you and then out of your attention.
   5. This is followed by the next thought that gently rises to the surface.

D. **Chakra Meditation**
   1. In chakra meditation, each of the seven **chakras** within the body corresponds with a specific color.
   2. These charkas become the point of focus.

E. **Walking Meditation**
   1. Walking meditation involves the use of movement as one's focus rather than a mantra or the breath.

VI. **BENEFITS OF MEDITATION**
A. During meditation, several physiological changes occur:
   1. Heartbeat and breathing rates slow down.
   2. Oxygen consumption falls by 20 percent.
   3. Blood lactate levels, which are known to rise with stress and fatigue, drop.
   4. Electroencephalograms (EEG) show an increase of alpha brain wave patterns, another sign of relaxation.
B. Many stress-related illnesses have also responded favorably to meditation:
   1. asthma, high blood pressure, heart disease, angina pectoris, serum cholesterol levels, insomnia, stuttering, diabetic conditions and depression.
   2. Fibromyalgia, headache pain, dementia caregiver stress, and anxiety.
C. Meditation has many psychological benefits including:
   1. Improved job performance and satisfaction
   2. Better academic performance in high school and college
   3. Increased long-term and short-term recall
   4. Sounder sleep
   5. Decreased anxiety
   6. Reduced fear
   7. Fewer phobias
   8. More positive mental health
D. Meditation can be seen as a useful and effective intervention in both reducing stress and dealing with a wide variety of stress-related illnesses.

VII. **FREQUENTLY ASKED QUESTIONS ABOUT MEDITATION**
A. How do I stay focused when I meditate?
   1. No matter what happens during meditation – staying focused on the mantra, scattered thinking, or falling asleep – you maintain one single intention when you meditate and that is to return to the mantra when it occurs to you to do so.
      a) There is no other effort involved.
B. When is the best time to meditate?
   1. Mornings and afternoons are best.
   2. When the stomach is mostly empty.
   3. Not before going to bed at night.
C. How long should I meditate?
   1. Any amount of time is good, but 15 to 20 minutes on as many days of the week as possible is optimum.
D. Will meditation get easier with practice?

    1. A person does not necessarily get better at meditation with regular practice any more than a person gets better at eating breakfast every day.
        a) The physiological and psychological effects of meditation tend to expand with practice.
        b) As meditation practice becomes regular, the effects of meditation remain throughout the day.
            (1) You feel calm and peaceful and enjoy all the benefits of feeling relaxed during the entire day.

  E. Does it really matter if I lie down, rather than sit, during meditation?
    1. It is best to practice meditation sitting rather than lying down.
        a) When you lie down, you tend to fall asleep during meditation.

  F. How will I know if I am getting the best results from meditation?
    1. The quality of a good meditation is not what happens during meditation.
    2. The quality of a good meditation is how you feel afterward.
        a) This is why it makes little difference what happens while you are meditating as long as you intend to return to your point of focus.
    3. How you feel afterwards is always the crucial determinant of whether or not the meditation is having positive effects for you.

VIII.   CONCLUSION
  A. While we may not entirely understand why meditation works so well or how it works, we know it works to enhance our health and well being.
  B. Simple meditation and breathing meditation are excellent techniques to get you started in experiencing the benefits of meditation.
  C. For those students who have learned meditation, there are few methods that are as warmly embraced for regaining balance, restoring energy, and bringing peace and tranquility.

LEARNING ACTIVITIES

ACTIVITY 1 - JOURNALING

Objective: The purpose of this activity is to encourage critical thinking and honest personal reflection on topics relating to the chapter content. Explore personal thoughts, feelings, values, and behaviors as you selectively incorporate stress management knowledge and behaviors into your plan for improved health through better stress management.

Instructions: You will find journaling questions in each chapter of your Activities Manual. These questions relate specifically to the chapter content. Moving your thoughts from your mind to the paper is a powerful strategy for relieving stress and for increasing awareness of your thoughts, feelings and behaviors. Your course instructor can provide further guidance on how to complete this activity.

Complete the following journaling questions. Select the questions that have the most relevance for you.

1. Try the activity under the heading 'What Meditation is Not'. What did you discover about your thoughts as you tried to eliminate them for 60 seconds?
2. What is a mantra? What might you choose for a personal mantra and why?
3. Why is it important to have a passive attitude during meditation?
4. How should you always end meditation and why is this so important?
5. What are three things that will commonly occur when you meditate? When any of these things happen, what should be your single intention?
6. What should be the test to determine if meditation is working for you?
7. Investigate Zen meditation. Check it out online or in the library and read about the underlying philosophy of Zen meditation. Think about how this style of meditation differs from the meditation styles presented in this chapter.
8. What are your beliefs about chakras? Do you believe that we could have energy flowing through our bodies and that this energy plays a part in our health?
9. How does the information in this chapter affect you personally? What insights did you have about yourself and the stress that you experience?

ACTIVITY 2 - RELAXATION EXERCISE - SIMPLE MEDITATION

Objectives: The purpose of this activity is to allow you to practice deep relaxation on your own using the relaxation exercise called Simple Meditation.

Materials needed:
Handout 21:1 - How to Meditate Using a Mantra
Handout 21:2 - Relaxation Exercise - Simple Meditation

Instructions:
1. Practice Simple Meditation at least two times on your own according to the instructions on the handout.

2. Assess your experiences with meditation using Handout 21:2 - Relaxation Exercise - Simple Meditation.

Handout 21:1 - How to Meditate Using a Mantra

The most important thing is don't try too hard. Don't make a big deal out of this. It is the easiest thing that our mind can do ... perhaps that is why it is so powerful.

1) Find a quiet environment where you won't be disturbed.

2) Sit comfortably **in a chair** (don't lie down) with the eyes closed. Try to be in a place with a minimum amount of noise and light but don't be too concerned with noises. They need not be a distraction to meditation. People have meditated in airports, in the car, in boring classes or meetings, and many other places. The important thing is to go through the process as described below.

3) Begin by sitting in your chair for about 30 seconds with the eyes closed and just get yourself in tune with your internal environment (do a quick body scan). Next, begin, as effortlessly and silently as possible repeating a word to yourself (not out loud). The word you choose is called a mantra.

   a. Examples of words (mantras) to use: still, one, relax, peace, empty, calm, serene, silent, tranquil, or any other word or phrase that is easy to remember (it makes no difference what word you use. It only matters that you proceed with the simple intention of repeating the word, over and over and over.).

   b. Simply repeat silently the mantra over and over to yourself.

   c. Just let your mind whisper your mantra under your thoughts, over and over and over. Don't try to change your thoughts in any way. Just allow yourself to keep whispering the word silently to yourself.

4) When you notice your mind wandering (it will) just notice it and gently bring your attention back to your breathing and your mantra. Don't think that you are a bad meditator if you don't remain with your word the entire time or even part of the time. The important thing is to gently return to the word when you catch your mind wandering... or falling asleep.

5) Practice for approximately 10-20 minutes every day (or at least 3-4 times per week). The best times to practice meditation are first thing in the morning and in the afternoon between 4 and 6 o'clock. To enhance your experience, try a little yoga just before meditating. A few sun salutes usually does the trick (See Chapter 22).

6) Don't think that this has to be any more difficult than it is explained here. There is nothing else to do besides silently repeat your mantra. Don't try to make anything happen. Just be present with your mantra. That's all! You only have one intention while you meditate: Return to your mantra when it occurs to you to do so. There is no other effort involved whatsoever.

7) Don't set an alarm clock but sit with a clock in view if necessary. It is okay to briefly open your eyes to check the time, then close them again and return to the mantra.

8) **Slowly** return to normal waking consciousness. Take at least 2 minutes to return. Don't be in a hurry or you will feel the same way you feel when an alarm clock or telephone awakens you out of a dream.

Several things might happen while you are meditating and each is entirely appropriate.

- You might easily repeat the mantra for the entire period that you are meditating. This is fine, but is not necessarily the goal. The goal is that you intend to repeat the word. Whether or not that happens is secondary.
- You might fall asleep. If you do, great. Enjoy it! You will probably have one of the deepest sleeps you have had in a while. Falling asleep while meditating is usually an indication that you need more sleep. You are giving yourself a perfect opportunity to catch up. When you do awaken from sleeping while meditating, be sure to spend a few more minutes going back to the mantra. Otherwise it will feel similar to the way that you feel when you are dreaming and you are abruptly awakened to a phone ringing or some other very jarring sound.
- Another thing that might happen is your mind will fly all over the place with thoughts. Don't be dismayed when this happens. Simply gently return to repeating the mantra. If the thoughts continue ceaselessly, simply intend to slip the mantra gently underneath the thoughts.
- Occasionally, but not very often, your mind will become very still. In that stillness, ideas, insights, perhaps we could call it inspiration or intuition will flood into your mind. Be sure to have a pen and paper ready to write down the interesting thoughts that come to you. Out of that silence sometimes comes exactly what we need to know or do as we progress on our path.

Remember, the quality of a good meditation is not what happens during the meditation. The important issue is how you feel after meditating. If you have more energy, more alertness, if your mind is calmer, more peaceful and you feel happier, this is feedback that your mind/body enjoys and finds benefit from the meditation.

Handout 21:2 - Relaxation Exercise
Simple Meditation

The relaxation homework assignment for this week is called Simple Meditation. Practice doing it the same way you did it in class.

Practice doing this exercise at least two times according to Handout 21:1 - How to Meditate Using a Mantra. Do it at times when you will not be disturbed. Try to spend about 15 minutes meditating on both occasions.

On your typed paper, *thoroughly* respond to each of these items referring to the two times that you did them at home, *and* the time that you did it in class. Describe primarily how you were feeling in relation to your stress levels.

Follow this general outline with your description:

Daytime (first time):
- How you felt before meditating
- Your ability to remain focused on your mantra
- What things you noticed were happening while you meditated (mental, emotional, physical)
- How you felt while you meditated
- How you felt after meditating (both immediately and for a while after meditating)
- Any other thoughts, concerns, or insights you had regarding your experience meditating

Daytime (second time):
- How you felt before meditating
- Your ability to remain focused on your mantra
- What things you noticed were happening while you meditated (mental, emotional, physical)
- How you felt while you meditated
- How you felt after meditating (both immediately and for a while after meditating)
- Any other thoughts, concerns, or insights you had regarding your experience meditating

Classroom experience (if applicable):
- How you felt before meditating
- Your ability to remain focused on your mantra
- What things you noticed were happening while you meditated (mental, emotional, physical)
- How you felt while you meditated
- How you felt after meditating (both immediately and for a while after meditating)
- Any other thoughts, concerns, or insights you had regarding your experience meditating

ACTIVITY 3 – MINI MEDITATION BREAK

Objectives: The purpose of this activity is to give you a quick relaxation break using a meditation technique.

Instructions: This activity can be done at any time of the day when you have a break in action and need a quick refresher.

Close your eyes while seated in a chair. Practice, for a brief period of time, one of the ways of meditating as outlined in chapter 21. Do this very mindfully—if your mind wanders, simply return your thoughts to your point of focus.

You don't need to do this for much longer than 5 minutes but any of the meditation techniques in chapter 21 can be done for any length of time.

RELATED WEBSITES

Meditation Station
Website on meditation by the Meditation Society of America
http://www.meditationsociety.com/

The TM program at a Glance
Background on Transcendental Meditation—the basis for the simple meditation exercise in chapter 21.
http://tm.org/discover/glance/index.html

TM—A Scientifically Validated Programme
A web page of research studies showing the effects of meditation
http://www.maharishi-india.org/programmes/p1tm.html

CHAPTER 22
YOGA

CHAPTER OUTLINE
Use this outline to take notes as you read the chapter in the text and/or as your instructor lectures in class.

I. **YOGA**
   A. **Yoga** is a course of exercises and postures intended to promote control of the body and mind and to attain physical and spiritual wellbeing.
   B. The term "yoga" comes from the Sanskrit root *yuj*, which means "to join" or "to yoke together."
      1. It literally signifies union of the body, mind, emotions and spirit into one harmonious and integrated whole.
   C. Yoga philosophy teaches ways of establishing harmony among the various sides of life.
      1. Once the mind and body have established harmony—have become integrated and still—healing happens at all levels.

II. **BACKGROUND**
   A. Yoga is said to have originated in India nearly 5,000 years ago.
      1. The tradition has been passed down from generation to generation by word of mouth, and from teacher to student.
   B. The **yoga sutras** (aphorisms or thoughts) have eight limbs or eight branches of yoga, including:
      1. **Yama**, meaning "restraint" — refraining from violence, lying, stealing, casual sex, and hoarding.
      2. **Niyama**, meaning "observance" — purity, contentment, tolerance, study, and remembrance.
      3. **Asana**, physical exercises.
      4. **Pranayama**, breathing techniques.
      5. **Pratyahara**, preparation for meditation, described as withdrawal of the mind from the senses.
      6. **Dharana**, concentration, being able to hold the mind on one object for a specified time.
      7. **Dhyana**, meditation, the ability to focus on one thing (or nothing) indefinitely.
      8. **Samadhi**, absorption, or realization of the essential nature of the self.
   C. Most yoga classes, books, and videos today focus on the third, fourth and fifth branches of yoga, namely asanas (postures or poses), pranayamas (breathing techniques), and pratyahara (meditation).
      1. Collectively, these three make up what is commonly known as **hatha yoga**.
   D. Yoga has no political or religious boundaries.
      1. Anyone can practice yoga regardless of age, sex, or physical condition.
      2. If a person is interested in beginning regular yoga practice, it is probably best to seek out a class with a qualified teacher who can provide guidance and instruction so that your initial experiences with yoga are positive ones.

III. **OVERVIEW OF YOGA STYLES**
   A. Hatha yoga focuses on simple poses that flow from one to the other at a very comfortable pace.
      1. Participants are encouraged to go at their own pace, taking time to focus on the breathing and meditation in their practice.
      2. This yoga is ideal for winding down at the end of a tough day.
   B. **Iyengar yoga** is a classical style of yoga that is softer on the body and is well-suited for beginners and those who haven't exercised in a while.
      1. It uses props such as chairs, straps, blocks, pillows, and sandbags to compensate for a lack of flexibility, which is helpful for anyone with back or joint problems.

C. **Ashtanga (power) yoga** is the preferred choice for athletes, since ashtanga yoga is light on meditation but heavy on developing strength and stamina.
    1. The poses are more difficult than those performed in other styles and students move quickly from one pose to another in an effort to build strength, stamina, and flexibility.
    2. The cornerstone of power yoga is the sun salutation.
D. **Kundalini yoga** incorporates mantras (chanting), meditations, visualizations, and guided relaxation.
    1. It focuses on healing and "purifying" the mind, body, and emotions.
E. **Bikram yoga** is done in a hot room that is 90 to 105 degrees Fahrenheit (to replicate the temperature of yoga's birthplace in India).
    1. This style of yoga moves sequentially through 26 postures that are performed in a precise order.
    2. The Bikram series warms and stretches muscles, ligaments and tendons in the order in which they should be stretched.
F. **Kripalu yoga** is more spontaneous, flowing, and meditation-orientated yoga.
    1. The essence of Kripalu yoga is experienced through a continuous flow of postures while meditating, for gentle yet dynamic yoga.
G. **Sivananda yoga** has a series of 12 poses, with the sun salutation, breathing exercises, relaxation, and mantra chanting as its foundation.

IV. WHAT IS HATHA YOGA?
A. Hatha yoga consists of regulation of the mind and body through 14 different breathing exercises (pranayamas), and over 200 balanced physical postures or poses (asanas) developed to exercise and lengthen all the muscles in the body.
    1. The physical postures involve learning to control, regulate, and become aware of one's physical existence.
        a) The emphasis is on giving complete mental attention to each movement, to the exclusion of everything else.
        b) With practice, different body functions become more integrated with one another with all parts functioning together harmoniously.
        c) Energy from within is awakened, and the person practicing yoga feels radiant with vitality and energy.
B. The practice of yoga postures (asanas) differs significantly from conventional exercise such as aerobics, weight training, and jogging.
    1. The goal of asana practice is to restore the mind-body to its natural condition of well-being, alertness, and potential peak performance.
    2. Developing muscle strength cardiovascular fitness and other health benefits are possible in the process but are commonly seen as secondary objectives.

V. BENEFITS OF YOGA
A. Regular practice of hatha yoga yields the following benefits:
    1. Better overall physical and mental health.
    2. Relieves and delays the onset of fatigue and makes up for lost sleep.
    3. Helps access and cultivate the skillful and healthy elements of the unconscious mind. This brings about a spiritual unfolding and leads to better mind-body integration and harmony and effortless living.
    4. Helps minimize and alleviate illusions, fatigue, confusion, inessential burdens and develops a living that is more skillful which allows us to let go of disturbing thoughts and feelings. It helps us deal with the life stresses we experience and brings about greater freedom from negative conditioning and repressed memories.
    5. Prepares the mind, body and breath for sitting concentration/meditation practice.

VI. HEALTH EFFECTS OF YOGA PRACTICE
A. Every symptom that occurs as a result of chronic activation of the stress response can be positively improved through regular practice of yoga.
    1. The American Yoga Association provides details of how yoga is helpful in alleviating

the symptoms of the following conditions: addiction, AIDS/HIV, anxiety and stress, arthritis, asthma, back and neck pain, chronic fatigue, depression, diabetes, fibromyalgia, headaches, heart health, hypertension, incontinence, infertility, insomnia, multiple sclerosis, pain management, PMS/menopause, and weight management.

    a) During yoga practice, the stress response turns off for the duration of the session.

        (1) As a result, the body functions that are altered when we perceive a need to run or fight return to homeostasis.

        (2) This balanced physiological state allows the body to correct problems that have occurred due to chronic stress for lasting results long after the yoga session has ended.

B. The asanas make use of gravity to increase blood flow to targeted areas.

C. Yoga poses increase flexibility in the spine.

D. The yoga postures stretch and relax muscles, increase flexibility in the joints, and stretch ligaments and tendons.

E. Asanas balance the nervous system.

    1. They increase flexibility, improve circulation, strengthen muscles, aid in digestion, improve the immune system, and improve breathing capacity and the elasticity of the lungs.

F. Yoga postures work on all dimensions of the mind-body:

    1. Physically, the body experiences healing, muscle strengthening, stretching and relaxation.

        a) All tissues and organs in the body get a workout, and even the nervous system returns to a more balanced state.

    2. Mentally, the mind cultivates peacefulness, alertness, and a heightened ability to focus and concentrate.

    3. Emotionally, yoga frees the mind from anxiety, worry, and tension and transforms negative emotions and behaviors into positive and higher states.

    4. Spiritually, yoga prepares one for meditation as it develops inner strength.

        a) Yoga experts claim that yoga helps an individual evolve spiritually as it enables him to understand and accept life's situations and experiences from a broader perspective, thereby increasing faith in a more elevated purpose, and in a higher power and the goodness of life.

    5. Behaviorally, yoga redirects wasted energy away from behaviors that could be detrimental to well-being.

VII. HOW TO PRACTICE YOGA

A. Yoga asanas are designed to develop the body with three primary aspects of fitness: power, flexibility, and balance.

    1. Every pose combines one or more of each of these aspects.

        a) Some poses may develop balance more than flexibility.

        b) Other poses are designed to develop strength and power.

    2. Working on a wide variety of poses develops each of these aspects of fitness throughout the entire body.

B. Asana practice for beginners and experienced yogis is essentially the same, the difference being the intensity of the poses and the flexibility of the student.

    1. In general, a typical yoga session consists of proceeding through a series of poses, being mindful of what is happening in the body, entering and ending each pose slowly, breathing fully and deeply in and out through the nose, and enjoying the process.

C. Yoga poses are done in a variety of positions including standing, sitting, kneeling, lying on the back, lying on the stomach, on the hands and knees, and in inverted positions.

    1. Each asana might have a number of variations.

    2. Depending on one's skill level, the poses may be modified to any of the variations.

        a) This is why yoga is appropriate for people of all levels of fitness and flexibility.

D. As you move into, and out of each pose, keep a part of the mind's focus on the flow of breathing.

   1. In general, inhalations take place during expansion phases of a pose; exhalations occur during the contracting phases of a pose.

      a) As a pose is held, allow the breath to flow like a circle going in through the nose, down into the lowest parts of the lungs, turning around and coming back out through the nose.

      b) Visualize the flowing breath like a moving Ferris wheel slowly moving around in a smooth circular pattern.

      c) There should be no jerkiness to the breath, nor should there be long pauses in the flowing breath between an inhale and exhale or between an exhale and inhale.

E. Move very slowly into and back out of each pose.

   1. Never jerk through a range of motion.

   2. Take your time and allow yourself to move smoothly from the beginning to the end of a pose.

      a) Hold each pose for at least 20 seconds; longer is better.

         (1) It takes about 20 seconds for the muscles, tendons, and ligaments to release and move into a stretching mode.

   3. There are some poses that involve movement rather than static stretching.

      a) Move through these movements slowly and easily.

F. Stretch to almost a maximal range of motion and then ease back just a little from there.

   1. This is where you start.

   2. As you are holding the pose, allow yourself to move ever so slightly more into the stretch each time you exhale.

      a) Let the exhale assist you in expanding.

   3. With practice you will find your body responding by easing you gently through your physical limits.

G. Keep your attention directly focused on what is happening in your body.

   1. Do not let your mind wander.

   2. As you maintain your focus, you can gently move through your limits and extend yourself while at the same time making sure that you are not overextending and causing unnecessary tissue damage.

   3. *Never push yourself through the range of a stretch to the point where you feel pain.*

      a) It's okay to have a feeling of slight muscle pulling, but pain is never a good thing when doing yoga.

         (1) If pain is felt, the tissue is sending a message that it is being pulled or pushed too far.

         (2) That leads to injuries and also creates a sensation of fear connected to that pose in the future.

H. Yoga is usually done barefoot, wearing comfortable athletic attire or loose clothing that breathes easily.

   1. Consider wearing what you wear when you go to the gym as appropriate for practicing yoga.

   2. You might find it helpful to bring a towel with you, and a yoga mat can be especially useful if the floor is hard.

   3. You can practice yoga nearly anywhere: at home, at school, in the office, at the beach, in a park, or anywhere you have some open space, peace and quiet, and some fresh air.

VIII.   **TIPS FOR ENHANCING YOUR YOGA EXPERIENCE**
    A. Try to do yoga on an empty stomach.
    B. You will experience benefits of yoga by practicing as little as one hour per week.
       1. The more you do it, the more you will experience the positive effects of yoga.
    C. When possible, try to practice at the same time every day.
    D. Go at your own pace.
       1. Don't compare your progress or your flexibility with anyone else.
    E. Take responsibility for your progress.
    F. Be patient with yourself.
       1. Don't look for immediate results.
       2. Release any and all expectations of how you *should* be progressing and simply let the experience of regular practice be sufficient.
    G. Enjoy the experience.
       1. Associate pleasure with stretching, breathing, and smooth body movement.
       2. Your body will tell you that this is a very healthy and useful thing to do.
       3. You will experience a flood of positive feelings both during and after yoga.

IX. **SAMPLE POSES**
    A. See Table 22:1 for demonstration of common yoga poses.
       1. Follow the principles outlined in this chapter as you practice the poses.

X. **CONCLUSION**
    A. Yoga signifies union of the body, mind, emotions, and spirit into one harmonious and integrated whole.
    B. Many styles and variations of yoga exist.
    C. Hatha yoga focuses on simple, flowing poses, along with breathing and meditation, making it especially effective for relaxation.
    D. Yoga postures work on all dimensions of the mind-body to activate the parasympathetic nervous system and initiate the relaxation response.

<u>LEARNING ACTIVITIES</u>

ACTIVITY 1 - JOURNALING

Objective: The purpose of this activity is to encourage critical thinking and honest personal reflection on topics relating to the chapter content. Explore personal thoughts, feelings, values, and behaviors as you selectively incorporate stress management knowledge and behaviors into your plan for improved health through better stress management.

Instructions: You will find journaling questions in each chapter of your Activities Manual. These questions relate specifically to the chapter content. Moving your thoughts from your mind to the paper is a powerful strategy for relieving stress and for increasing awareness of your thoughts, feelings and behaviors. Your course instructor can provide further guidance on how to complete this activity.

Complete the following journaling questions. Select the questions that have the most relevance for you.

1. Why do you think yoga works to decrease activation of the stress response?
2. How have your perceptions of yoga changed since you read this chapter and practiced doing some of the poses?
3. Without knowing too much about yoga, which of the yoga styles might best fit your personal levels of fitness, flexibility and interest? Explain why you feel this way.
4. Describe the positive health effects of yoga that are the most interesting to you.
5. Which poses did you feel were most difficult? Easiest? Most relaxing?
6. Expound on three of the listed Tips for Enhancing your Yoga Experience.
7. How does the information in this chapter affect you personally? What insights did you have about yourself and the stress that you experience?

ACTIVITY 2 - RELAXATION EXERCISE - YOGA

Objectives: The purpose of this activity is to allow you to practice yoga on your own.

Materials needed:
Handout 22:1 - Yoga Assessment
Handout 22:2 - Yoga Practice
Chapter 22 of the textbook (especially Table 22.1 Common Yoga Poses)

Instructions:
1. Practice Yoga at least two times on your own according to the instructions on Handout 22:2 - Yoga Practice.

2. Complete Handout 22:1 - Yoga Assessment.

Handout 22:1 – Yoga Assessment

Your Name _____

1. In a few sentences, write how you felt *while we went through the yoga poses*. Describe your experience.

2. In a few sentences, describe how you felt *after we finished the yoga* (both immediately after and for the few hours that followed).

3. In what ways, if any, have your perceptions and understandings changed about yoga since learning about it and practicing it?

Handout 22:2 - Yoga Practice

On 2 separate occasions during this week experiment with 10 different poses according to the instructions and poses in the text. Choose at least ten per session and do them exactly as they are pictured in the text.

Follow the guidelines, tips and pointers for proper yoga in chapter 22 of your text as you do these. Among those that you do, try the following simple poses:

- Standing forward bend
- Triangle pose I
- Thunderbolt
- Downward Dog
- Child's pose I
- Head to the Knee
- Spinal Twist
- Bridge
- Belly Turning pose
- Sun Salute (Be sure to follow this carefully as it is a series of sequential poses.)
- Corpse pose (always end with this one)

It may help to copy the instructions and print them out or work with a partner.

Realize that there are an enormous number of poses. These are just a few common ones and a great start to a life of great yoga.

In a typed format, please answer the following questions in relation to your practice:

1. Which poses did you choose each time?
2. Which did you find difficult, easy, or impossible?
3. How did you feel before, during and after doing the yoga sessions?
4. After actually doing yoga, describe how your perceptions have changed. How did you perceive yoga before?

ACTIVITY 3 –YOGA ON THE WEB

The ideal way to learn yoga is by going to a yoga class or by one-on-one instruction. Next best is to be shown examples of yoga and then try them on your own by watching a video or television. The Internet is another good way to discover more about yoga.

There are many places on the web to learn more about yoga. A great overview of yoga can be found by going to this website:

http://healthology.com/search.asp?keyword=yoga

Once there, click on the first listing titled "An Introduction to Yoga." You will get a "webcast" of an interview between an interviewer and 2 people who are talking about yoga. If you can't get the webcast (due to limitations of your computer), you can view the transcript.

This is a nice overview of yoga. It answers many questions people have who have never encountered yoga before, but have an interest in learning more about it.

Two additional useful websites for basic and advanced information on yoga can be found at:

http://www.santosha.com/asanas/

http://www.yogajournal.com/poses/index.cfm?ctsrc=hg7

What new ideas did you gain from exploring these sites?

RELATED WEBSITES

Step-by-Step Yoga Postures
An online resource for the practice of yoga postures
http://www.santosha.com/asanas/

YogaJournal—Yoga poses
Use the search tools to find asanas (poses) by anatomical focus, therapeutic application, or contraindication or just browse poses by name.
http://www.yogajournal.com/poses/index.cfm?ctsrc=hg7

Introduction to Yoga
Click the words "Introduction to Yoga" to hear a webcast that overviews yoga.
http://healthology.com/search.asp?keyword=yoga

CHAPTER 23
COMPLEMENTARY AND ALTERNATIVE HEALTH

CHAPTER OUTLINE
Use this outline to take notes as you read the chapter in the text and/or as your instructor lectures in class.

I. **COMPLEMENTARY AND ALTERNATIVE HEALTH**
    A. **Complementary and alternative medicine** (CAM) is a group of diverse medical and health care systems, practices, and products that are not presently considered part of conventional medicine.
        1. Many of these practices have been used successfully throughout history and in cultures around the world to promote balance and well-being.
        2. The list of what is considered to be CAM changes continually, as those therapies that are proven to be safe and effective become adopted into conventional health care and as new approaches to health care emerge.
II. **UNDERSTANDING COMPLEMENTARY AND ALTERNATIVE HEALTH**
    A. **Complementary medicine** is used together with conventional medicine.
    B. **Alternative medicine** is used in place of conventional medicine.
    C. **Integrative medicine** combines mainstream medical therapies and CAM therapies.
    D. A common aspect of nearly every CAH practice is the component of balance.
    E. 36 percent of U.S. adults aged 18 years and over use some form of complementary and alternative medicine.
        1. When prayer specifically for health reasons is included in the definition of CAM, the number of U.S. adults using some form of CAM in the past year rises to 62 percent.
III. **CATEGORIES OF COMPLEMENTARY AND ALTERNATIVE MEDICINE**
    A. NCCAM classifies CAM therapies into five categories, or domains:
        1. Alternative Medical Systems - Examples include homeopathic medicine, naturopathic medicine, traditional Chinese medicine, and ayurveda.
        2. Mind-Body Interventions - Examples include meditation, prayer, mental healing, biofeedback and therapies that use creative outlets such as art, music, or dance.
        3. Biological-Based Therapies - Examples include dietary supplements and herbal products.
        4. Energy Therapies - Include two types; **biofield therapies** and **bioelectromagnetic-based therapies.** Examples of energy therapies include qi gong, reiki, therapeutic touch and the unconventional use of electromagnetic fields.
        5. Manipulative and Body-Based Methods - Examples include chiropractic or osteopathic manipulation and massage.
IV. **APPLICATIONS OF THE FIVE CATEGORIES OF CAM TO STRESS MANAGEMENT**
    A. Alternative Medical Systems
        1. **Traditional Chinese Medicine** includes carefully formulated techniques such as acupuncture, herbal medicine, massage, qi gong, and nutrition.
        2. **Ayurveda** is India's traditional system of natural medicine and is claimed to be the oldest system of natural healing on earth.
            a) An integral component of ayurvedic medicine is teaching people how to release stress and tension through the practice of meditation and yoga.
            b) Ayurveda believes that all aspects of life contribute to health, including nutrition, hygiene, sleep, weather, and lifestyle, as well as physical, mental, and sexual activities.
            c) Emotional factors are also taken into consideration. Anger, fear, anxiety, and unhealthy relationships are believed to contribute to illness.
            d) A healthy emotional state is considered the very foundation of physical health.

3. **Naturopathic medicine** - Modern naturopathy is founded on six basic principles:
   a) Nature has the power to heal. The physician's role is to support the self-healing process by removing obstacles to health.
   b) Treat the whole person. Disease rarely has a single cause, so every aspect of the patient must be brought into harmonious balance.
   c) First, do no harm. A physician should use methods and substances that are as nontoxic and noninvasive as possible.
   d) Identify and treat the cause. Rather than suppress symptoms, the physician should treat the underlying causes of disease.
   e) Prevention is as important as cure. A physician should help create health, as well as cure disease.
   f) Doctors should be teachers. Part of the physician's task is to educate the patient and encourage self-responsibility.

B. Mind-Body Interventions
   1. **Biofeedback** is especially valuable for stress-related conditions.
   2. Since the 1970s, empirical research has demonstrated that humans can gain control over several autonomic nervous system functions such as heart rate, blood pressure, salivation and skin temperature.

C. Biological-Based Therapies
   1. Ongoing research explores the connection between natural substances, such as herbs, dietary supplements and vitamins, and stress and anxiety relief.
   2. While there is often compelling evidence that the products are effective for inducing relaxation, adequate studies have often not been conducted to determine such things as potential side-effects or contraindications with other drugs.

Energy Therapies
   1. Energy therapies involve the use of energy fields including **meridians**, invisible channels of energy that flow in the body, or energy fields outside the body.
      a) In Chinese healing theory, each person has flowing through their body a vital energy that called *chi* (also called qi) that sustains life and from which all other activities flow.
      b) The chi flows through the body by way of meridians.
      c) When a person has a sickness or diseases, the underlying cause of the problem is thought to be a blockage of this flowing energy through the meridians.
      d) Some techniques, such as reflexology, acupressure, acupuncture, and shiatsu combine energy balance with massage.
   2. **Reflexology** is based on a system of points in the hands and feet that are believed to correspond to all areas of the body.
      a) Because each zone or part of the body has a corresponding reflex point on the feet, stimulating that reflex point causes restoration of the natural energy of the related organ.
   3. **Acupuncture** involves inserting hair-thin, sterile needles into the body at specific points (acupoints) to manipulate the body's flow of energy to balance the endocrine system.
   4. **Acupressure** is often described as acupuncture without the needles.
   5. **Shiatsu** means "finger pressure" in Japanese and is a synthesis of acupuncture and traditional Japanese massage.
   6. Acupuncture, acupressure, and shiatsu are intended to open the flow of chi, restore balance and support the natural healing of the body.
      a) Feelings of deep relaxation and increased vitality are common benefits of these treatments.
   7. Four additional energy therapies are **qi gong, tai chi, therapeutic touch,** and **reiki.**

E. Manipulative and Body-Based Methods
  1. The purpose of massage is to work on tension-packed muscles, to relax the muscles directly by pressure and rubbing.
  2. Massage is known to be effective in relieving stress related symptoms at the physical, mental and emotional level.
  3. Several types of massage work to relax the muscles in different ways.
    a) **Swedish massage** affects nerves, muscles, glands, and circulation, and promotes health and well-being.
    b) **Deep tissue massage** is used to release the chronic patterns of tension in the body through deep muscle compression with the heel of the hand, the pads of the thumb, and even the elbow pressing deliberately along the grain of the muscle
    c) **Myotherapy** targets trigger points that are diffused or erased by concentrated pressure applied to the trigger points for a short period of time (several seconds to two or three minutes) by the fingers, knuckles and elbows.
    d) **Craniosacral therapy** (CST) is a gentle, hands-on method of evaluating and enhancing the function of a physiological body system called the craniosacral system.
    e) **Sports massage** is a special type of massage focusing on muscle systems specific to athletics and sports.
    f) **Chair massage**, also known as on-site massage or corporate massage is administered while the person receiving the massage is fully clothed and seated in a specially designed chair.
    g) **Hot stone massage**, commonly used in health spas, uses stones that are heated and positioned on specific locations on the body. The stones are gently moved to other locations on the body with the light pressure being applied directly to the stones.

V. CONCLUSION
  A. As the research continues and as the public increasingly uses these techniques, complementary and alternative therapies will take an expanded role in stress management and health promotion.
  B. Research indicates that many forms of CAM are very effective, especially for preventing stress-related conditions and for promoting balance and well-being.
  C. You must take responsibility to investigate what is acceptable, safe and effective for you.
    1. Experiment with those therapies that seem interesting and feasible to you and discover some options for stress management and health that may seem new and unusual.
  D. People around the world, for generations, have found that they work.

LEARNING ACTIVITIES

ACTIVITY 1 – JOURNALING

Objective: The purpose of this activity is to encourage critical thinking and honest personal reflection on topics relating to the chapter content. Explore personal thoughts, feelings, values, and behaviors as you selectively incorporate stress management knowledge and behaviors into your plan for improved health through better stress management.

Instructions: You will find journaling questions in each chapter of your Activities Manual. These questions relate specifically to the chapter content. Moving your thoughts from your mind to the paper is a powerful strategy for relieving stress and for increasing awareness of your thoughts, feelings and behaviors. Your course instructor can provide further guidance on how to complete this activity.

Complete the following journaling questions. Select the questions that have the most relevance for you.

1. What is your perception of our traditional Western medicine health system, including its strengths and weakness in dealing with problems like stress-related disease? Compare and contrast the Western medicine approach to stress management with one of the alternative medical systems explained in this chapter.
2. What do you think of the use of medication to control stress? Do some research on the types of medications used for treating stress-related problems. What is your opinion on how health professionals approach treatment for stress?
3. Groucho Marx commented, "Be open-minded, but not so open-minded that your brains fall out." Explain how his comment might relate to alternative and complementary therapies. Of the therapies and techniques explained in this chapter, which would you consider using for stress management?
4. How does the information in this chapter affect you personally? What insights did you have about yourself and the stress that you experience?

ACTIVITY 2 – EXPERIENCING MASSAGE

Objectives: The purpose of this activity is to provide you with the experience of giving and receiving massage.

Materials needed:
Handout 23:1 – Massage Assessment

Instructions:
Using the information provided in class and from your textbook, practice both giving and receiving a massage. You can do this at home or as a class activity. Your instructor will provide instructions for the in-class activity.

Handout 23:1 – Massage Assessment

Your Name _____

1. In a few sentences, write how you felt while you *received* the massage. Describe your experience.

2. In a few sentences, write how you felt while you *gave* the massage. Describe your experience.

3. In a few sentences, describe how you felt after you finished getting a massage (both immediately after and for the few hours that followed).

4. In what ways, if any, have your perceptions and understandings changed about massage since learning about it and practicing it in class?

ACTIVITY 3 – COMPLEMENTARY/ALTERNATIVE THERAPY ARTICLE DAY

Objectives: The purpose of this activity is to raise awareness about a wide variety of complementary and alternative therapies that are available.

Instructions:
Find a study or article and write a brief, double-spaced, typed summary of the article that should answer the following questions:
- What motivated you to select this article about this particular alternative therapy?
- What were the main points of the article?
- What did you learn about the complementary/alternative therapy that you didn't know before?
- How does the therapy relate to stress management?
- What are your personal feelings about the article? How did it affect you? Did it motivate you to change anything about your lifestyle? For example, would you consider adopting the type of therapy for yourself?
- What other thoughts did you have as you were reading this article?

Include a photocopy of the actual article complete with the reference page(s) at the end of the article. This photocopied article should be stapled to the summary of the article.

The following is a list of possible topics from which you can choose your article. Be sure your review explains how your topic relates to stress and/or stress management. For instance, if you choose acupuncture, your paper will need to be about a connection between stress and acupuncture. If you choose music, it will need to discuss the relationship between music and stress.

Aromatherapy	Ayurveda	Biofeedback
Bodywork	Breathwork	Chinese Medicine
Colonic Cleansing	Color Therapy	Art Therapy
Flower Essences	Gemstone Therapy	Herbs, Roots, & Seeds
Homeopathy	Iridology	Macrobiotics
Hypnosis	Acupuncture	Therapeutic Humor
Massage	Massage Therapy	Reiki
Music Therapy	Naturopathy	Polarity Therapy
Qigong	Magnets	Tai chi
Sensory Deprivation	Therapeutic Touch	Yoga

ACTIVITY 4 – COMPLEMENTARY/ALTERNATIVE HEALTHCARE PRACTITIONER INTERVIEW

Objectives: The purpose of this activity is to provide you with an opportunity to interview a complementary practitioner. This helps you differentiate between traditional and complementary/alternative approaches to healthcare and increases your awareness of the strengths and weaknesses of different approaches to dealing with health issues such as stress.

Materials needed:
Handout 23:2 – Practitioner Interview

Instructions: Follow the directions on Handout 23:2 – Practitioner Interview. Be sure to plan ahead on scheduling the interview. Professionals that can be interviewed include practitioners of massage, chiropractics, acupuncture, herbal therapies, therapeutic touch, reiki, meditation, naturopathy, homeopathy, and many other therapies.

Handout 23:2 – Practitioner Interview

Directions: *Make an appointment well in advance of the assignment due date to interview a complementary health care practitioner. Explain that you are taking this class and explain the purpose of this assignment. Remember that these are busy professionals so be organized and appreciative of the time they spend with you. As a courtesy, consider sending a follow up thank you note.*

Submit a 1-2 page typed report based on your interview with a complementary/alternative healthcare provider including the information listed below.

Practitioner Name and Credentials:

Job Title and Worksite Location:

Years of experience:

Date of Interview:

1. Describe how you became interested in the complementary therapy/intervention you practice.

2. Describe the types of clients who seek your services. Are your services covered by insurance?

3. Describe your working relationship with traditional health care providers (Medical doctors, nurse practitioners, physical therapists, etc.). Do you refer clients to them? Do they refer clients to you?

4. Explain your education & training.

5. Explain your philosophy of health care.

6. In your opinion, what impact does stress have on the health of the patients/clients who seek your services?

Students: After you have completed the interview, reflect back on what you learned. Your report will include the answers to the questions above and a one-two paragraph summary of what you learned from this assignment.

RELATED WEBSITES

National Center for Complementary and Alternative Medicine
Extensive website on nearly all aspects of CAM
http://nccam.nih.gov/

Traditional Chinese Medicine
An Alternative and Complementary Medicine Resource Guide
http://www.amfoundation.org/tcm.htm

What Is Biofeedback?
Excellent overview of biofeedback as a method for voluntarily decreasing parasympathetic nervous system activity.
http://www.psychotherapy.com/bio.html

CHAPTER 24
MORE STRESS REDUCTION STRATEGIES

CHAPTER OUTLINE
Use this outline to take notes as you read the chapter in the text and/or as your instructor lectures in class.

I. MORE STRESS-REDUCTION STRATEGIES
   A. This chapter looks at a smorgasbord of additional ways to reduce stress, though they may not initially be considered for that purpose.
   B. They are things that we commonly include in our lives that, by their nature, can make us feel better.
   C. While some of these stress reduction methods have not been as thoroughly examined scientifically, strong anecdotal evidence supports their effectiveness.
   D. The best attitude for the approaches described in this chapter is that of discovery.
      1. Experiment with the strategies and see which ones work for you.
      2. If you are like most people, you will find positive results as you incorporate several into your lifestyle and daily activities.

II. LAUGHTER & HUMOR
   A. The saying that laughter is good medicine has proven to be true. **Humor** differs from laughter in that a sense of humor is a learned, intellectual process. **Sarcasm** is the darker side of humor and is often used to put people down.
   B. **Laughter** can help prevent stress and has positive health benefits.
      1. The pleasant feelings associated with laughter may modify some of the neuroendocrine components of the stress response.
      2. Stress hormones that constrict blood vessels and suppress immune activity decrease after being exposed to humor.
   C. Laughter creates predictable physiological changes in the body in a manner similar to exercise.
      1. The arousal phase, with an increase in physiological measures like pulse, respirations, and blood pressure.
      2. The resolution phase, during which physiological measures return to resting values or lower values, creating a relaxation response.
   D. Laughter creates the positive stress known as eustress.
   E. Laughter is associated with a release of tension and an increase in the natural mood-lifters known as endorphins.
      1. **Endorphins** are mood elevating, pain-relieving chemicals produced naturally by the brain.
   F. Humor can also empower people by giving them a different perspective on life's problems.
   G. Subjective nature of humor - What makes us laugh is different for different individuals.
      1. What is important is to find ways to laugh every day.

III. MUSIC
   A. Music creates the mood for many settings.
   B. Music has been used throughout history to calm body, mind, and spirit. **Music therapy** applies the healing power of music and has been recorded in history as far back as biblical times.
   C. Clinical studies and anecdotal evidence from music therapists to conclude that music helps to:
      1. Manage pain
      2. Improve mood and mobility
      3. Reduce the need for pain relievers and sedatives accompanied with surgery
      4. Relieve anxiety
      5. Lower blood pressure

6. Ease depression
7. Enhance concentration and creativity
8. Certain kinds of music have been found to lower heart rates, respiratory rates, blood pressure, and increase tranquil mood states, regulate heart and breathing rate, and increase oxygen levels in the blood.
9. For individuals with hypertension and related conditions, music can be included with other therapies to promote health.

D. Here are findings from other studies:
1. Surgical patients exposed to music reported significantly lower pain intensity and required less morphine compared to a control group.
2. Subjects with osteoarthritis reported less arthritic pain when music was played compared to a control group who simply sat quietly.
3. People undergoing surgery have been shown to require fewer anesthesias, awaken from anesthesia more quickly and with fewer side effects, and heal more rapidly when healing music is played before, during, and after the surgical procedure.
4. Individuals suffering from depression need less medication and have more success in psychotherapy when music is added to their course of treatment.
5. Grief, loneliness, and anger are all managed better when appropriate music is added to therapy.
6. Autistic children and children diagnosed with brain damage all react positively to music therapy.

E. Music can affect the body and mind in two distinct ways:
1. Directly, as the effect of sound upon the cells and organs. **Medical resonance therapy music** is based on the underlying principle that music can influence our body directly at the cellular and organ level.
2. Indirectly, by affecting the emotions, which in turn influence numerous bodily processes.

F. What is the best type of music for reducing stress or for helping create a relaxing environment?
1. **Classical music** is one of the best types of music for relaxation and meditation.
   a) One type of early classical music that appears to be the most effective in reducing the stress response is music from the baroque period.
      (1) **adagio movements** of the baroque and early classical compositions, with a tempo of about 60 beats per minute appeared to be the most relaxing and produced heightened levels of alpha brainwave activity similar to what occurs during deep relaxation, hypnosis, and meditation.
      (2) The music of Mozart has become so popular as a healing tool that the treatment has become known as the **Mozart effect**.
2. **New Age music** is another genre that has become a well-accepted and effective type of music for stress management.
   a) New Age music does not mainly build on the principle of tension and release (like most music in general) but rather functions like wall paper, (meaning it just rests quietly and almost unnoticed in the background) which can create a positive, even healing atmosphere.

IV. **WHAT ELSE CAN I DO?**
A. Listen to your body
1. Tune in to signals like fatigue, headache, muscle pain, irritability and many more and become familiar with the ones that occur most frequently in you.
2. If you notice a headache beginning each time you feel overwhelmed, this is a signal to you that your stress response is up and running in high gear.
3. Pay attention to the other signals that your body gives you during tense times.
4. At the onset of these symptoms, do something to immediately reduce the stress you are feeling so you can deal with the situation appropriately, without the

additional false sense of alarm.

B. Deal directly with the cause
   1. Narrow down your stressors specifically and determine if there is something you can do to eliminate or modify the most stressful ones.

C. Distance yourself
   1. A time-out can effectively be used as a tool to help someone step out of a stressful situation, cool down, and refocus on what is really important.
   2. From an emotional distance, it's sometimes easier to see the situation more clearly and act appropriately.

D. Talk yourself through a situation
   1. Instead of saying, I'll never get this done in time," say, "I've been in similar situations before and managed it all right!"
   2. Be your own cheerleader; give yourself pep talks instead of self-scoldings.

E. Pat yourself on the back
   1. When you are successful at something, take a moment to allow yourself to feel good about a job well done.
      a) Curiously, we are quick to negatively judge our actions when we think we haven't measured up.
      b) Why not choose the opposite route when we have successfully made the grade?

F. Be creative
   1. When you are in a stressful situation, take a few minutes to write down every possible solution to the problem, regardless of how impossible or crazy it might seem.
   2. Writing your list of options reminds you that you do have the freedom to select your course of action, you do have some control.

G. Change your attitude
   1. Anytime you catch yourself thinking or saying that something is a problem, change how you think and speak of it by calling it a challenge.
      a) Challenges are viewed differently than problems.

H. Keep agreements
   1. When we keep agreements, things work out; the systems in which we live run smoothly.
   2. We also maintain our integrity when we keep agreements.
   3. When we don't keep agreements, things do not run as smoothly and integrity is lost.

I. Take short naps
   1. Naps are short periods of rest that recharge the body for the remainder of the day.
   2. Short Naps Are Best
      a) Researchers have found that a brief afternoon nap of only ten minutes was more recuperative than a thirty-minute nap in terms of improved alertness and performance in the hour following napping.

J. Change your physiology; change your feelings
   1. We can change how we are feeling by changing how our body is positioned, how it moves, how we speak as well as the things that we focus our thinking on.
   2. It is possible to trick our emotions into feeling better by putting our body into the position that it usually feels when we are happy, energized, and alive.
      a) Curiously, emotions will follow the body's physiology.
   3. A smart way to change your physiology, and thereby change how you feel, is by exercising.

K. Write about it
   1. Keeping a diary, or **journaling**, is a proven way for releasing our emotions by writing them.
   2. Keeping a stress diary can help you identify stressors in your life.

        a) Once identified, these stressors can be more easily managed.

        b) Giving yourself a few minutes to put your thoughts into words may be effective in helping you deal with the problem at hand.

L. Talk it out
1. Sometimes discussing problems with a trusted friend can help clear your mind so you can concentrate on problem solving.
    a) Learning to talk things over with someone you trust can release the pressure, make you feel better, and help you come to a new understanding of the problem.

M. Cry it out
1. We can find relief from stress by physically releasing these emotions.
    a) Sometimes crying is the best way to do this.
2. Many people report feeling relief after releasing pent-up emotions by crying it out.

N. Scream it out
1. Similar to crying, the act of releasing pent-up energy by loud verbal emissions or screaming has been found to be a useful way to release emotional energy for many people.
2. This can be done by just turning up the radio in your car and singing your favorite song at the top of your lungs or putting your face into your pillow and blasting away with all your might.

O. Sing it out
1. Many people relax by playing their favorite instrument.
2. Singing may also be a relaxing way to relieve stress.
    a) People sing in the shower, while driving, or while doing chores.
3. Many people add music to make work less stressful.

P. Dance it out
1. The combined benefits of exercise and music can come together in a fun and relaxing way when we dance to relieve stress.

Q. Focus on the needs of others
1. Taking attention from our own problems and shifting it to the needs of someone else tends to help us forget about the rough times we are going through.
    a) As people see the challenges others are facing, they often gain a new perspective on their own challenges.
    b) They develop an attitude of gratitude instead of self-pity.
    c) They also feel fulfillment from helping others in need.

R. Have sex
1. The physiological experience of the sexual response typically has a relaxing effect on the body and mind.
    a) During the orgasm phase of the sexual response, many muscles throughout the body tense.
    b) Following orgasm, those tensed muscles automatically relax. This leaves the body feeling deeply relaxed.

S. Soak in the tub
1. The warmth of the water is relaxing to the muscles.
    a) Being by yourself without anything else to do except enjoy the water is relaxing as well.
    b) As a pleasant way to unwind after a rough day, try placing lit aromatic candles around the bathtub.
    c) Soak in warm water with relaxing music playing and let the peaceful environment and soothing warm water completely relax the body and mind.

T. Gaze at the sky
1. Pondering the vastness of the universe can make many problems seem insignificant.
2. Enjoy the constant changes in the atmosphere.

3. Realize that the sky is perfect in every way, yet it is always changing.
   a) Consider this as a good metaphor for your own life.

U. Remember, it's the little things that add up
   1. Each individual stressor that we experience can work together with the others to produce a large mountain of stress.
   2. Viewed on the positive side, immersing ourselves in many small positive things can also add up to a large contribution toward a more relaxing lifestyle.
      a) View the list of "little things" that are included here in the text.

V. "SOLUTIONS" TO AVOID
   A. Gossip
      1. Spreading negative thoughts creates and intensifies negative feelings and emotions.
      2. There may be a short-term pleasurable feeling, but in the long run, gossip creates negative social and emotional problems as well as feelings of guilt.
   B. Whine and complain
      1. Whining doesn't deal with the problem directly, but makes the problem seem bigger than it really is by expanding it in the mind.
      2. Nobody enjoys being around someone who is constantly telling everyone how bad things are by vying for sympathy or pity for their problems.
   C. Blame others
      1. Blaming someone else for the consequences of your actions merely shows an unwillingness to accept responsibility for who and where you are.
      2. If you don't accept responsibility, then you also deny yourself the power to change or to make things better.
   D. Self-inflict pain
      1. Sometimes we may already feel severe emotional pain because of various emotional traumas like abuse or neglect.
         a) One way that some people choose to try to deal with that emotional distress is by creating a physical pain to release it.
      2. Experiencing a physical pain to try to drown the emotional distress may work in the short term, but as an alternate method of managing stress it is ineffective because of added emotional stresses it causes like guilt, shame and embarrassment.
      3. If this is used as a method to cope with emotional distress, the best solution may be to get help from a counselor or licensed therapist.
   E. Overdo it
      1. Any activity that is healthy in moderation becomes unhealthy and leads to more stress when it is overdone.
      2. How do we tell if we are overdoing something?
      3. Our body and mind will give us feedback that indicates that we are overdoing it.
         a) If we don't feel well after we are finished, if we are not living according to our highest values, if we are ignoring important things in life, if we feel uneasy or apathetic, we need to see these signals as feedback that we are overdoing something.
   F. Attempt suicide
      1. Attempting suicide indicates that a person believes he or she has run out of options.
         a) Suicide eliminates all other possibilities and devastates family members and friends.
         b) If you are considering suicide as a way to deal with your stress, get help.
            (1) Even if you don't think anyone else could possibly assist you, there are answers to every problem.

VI. CONCLUSION

A. Whichever methods of stress reduction you choose to include is up to you, but feel confident that you now have a tool chest full of stress-relievers.

B. Your personality and the situations in which you find yourself will determine which tools will work most effectively for you.

C. With practice, the tools become sharper and you will be more proficient at handling the stressors with which you are dealing.

   1. As you use these tools, you will find yourself calmer, more peaceful, and less likely to get upset when disturbing things happen.

<u>LEARNING ACTIVITIES</u>

ACTIVITY 1 - JOURNALING

Objective: The purpose of this activity is to encourage critical thinking and honest personal reflection on topics relating to the chapter content. Explore personal thoughts, feelings, values, and behaviors as you selectively incorporate stress management knowledge and behaviors into your plan for improved health through better stress management.

Instructions: You will find journaling questions in each chapter of your Activities Manual. These questions relate specifically to the chapter content. Moving your thoughts from your mind to the paper is a powerful strategy for relieving stress and for increasing awareness of your thoughts, feelings and behaviors. Your course instructor can provide further guidance on how to complete this activity.

Complete the following journaling questions. Select the questions that have the most relevance for you.

1. Which types of music do you find most relaxing? What is it about that type of music that you find so enjoyable?
2. What stressful situations might you be dealing with in your life right now, which, if you tried to look at the funny side of them, would make the situations seem less stressful?
3. When you want to get something "off your chest," do you find that it works best for you to talk, cry, scream, write it out on paper, or some combination of these? How do you think this works?
4. Look over the list of options in the "What Else Can I Do?" section of this chapter. Pick the three choices that would be most beneficial to you and write how you could incorporate them into your daily routines.
5. Think of a time when you helped someone else out, a time when you attended to the needs of another person. How did you find yourself feeling about your own cares, concerns, and worries as you performed this service?
6. Just as the little things add up on the negative side, how do you think little positive things can add up to a life with far less stress?
7. How does the information in this chapter affect you personally? What insights did you have about yourself and the stress that you experience?

ACTIVITY 2 – RELAXATION EXERCISE – GUIDED IMAGERY
FLOATING THROUGH COLORS

Objectives: The purpose of this activity is to allow you to practice deep relaxation using the Guided Imagery - Floating through Colors relaxation exercise.

Materials needed:
Stress Relief DVD
Handout 24:1 - DVD Relaxation Exercise – Guided Imagery - Floating through Colors

Instructions:
1. Practice Guided Imagery - Floating through Colors at least two times on your own.
   2. Assess your experience of this activity using Handout 24:1 - DVD Relaxation Exercise - Guided Imagery - Floating through Colors.

Handout 24:1 - DVD Relaxation Exercise
Guided Imagery – Floating through Colors

The DVD homework assignment for this week is the seventh exercise on the Stress Relief DVD called "Guided Imagery – Floating through Colors."

Practice doing this exercise at least two (2) times according to the instructions on the DVD.

Do it at times when you will not be disturbed. It lasts approximately 15 minutes.

In a *typed* format, respond to the following items:

1. How you felt before the exercise
2. Your experience during the exercise
3. How you felt immediately following the exercise
4. How you felt long after completing the exercise

On your typed paper, ***thoroughly*** respond to each of these items referring to the two times that you did them at home, *and* the time that you did it in class. Describe primarily how you were feeling in relation to your stress levels.

Follow this general outline with your description:

Daytime (first time):
- Before
- During
- Immediately after
- Long after

Daytime (second time):
- Before
- During
- Immediately after
- Long after

Classroom experience (if applicable):
- Before
- During
- Immediately after
- Long after

ACTIVITY 3 – HUMOR HEALTH EFFECTS – INTERNET ACTIVITY

Objectives: The purpose of this activity is to give you more information on the positive benefits of humor from an internet website.

Materials needed:
Internet access to the following website:

http://www.jesthealth.com/artantistress.html

Instructions:
Go to the website and review it. In your own words (using your word processor) summarize the following aspects of humor based on what you read:

- Historical perspective of humor
- Effect of humor on the spirit
- Norman Cousins' thoughts on humor
- Effect of humor on the body
- Effect of humor on the mind
- Your thoughts about this article

ACTIVITY 4 – FUNNY MOVIE

Objectives: The purpose of this activity is to give you a break from all things serious by enjoying your favorite humorous movie.

Instructions:
Complete this activity by viewing again the funniest movie you have ever seen, just for the health of it.

Write a brief paper about your experience: Which movie you chose, why you chose the movie, what it was about the movie that was so humorous, and how your stress level changed as a result of watching the movie.

ACTIVITY 5- RELAXING MUSIC

Objectives: The purpose of this activity is to introduce you to relaxing music as discussed in Chapter 24 of the text.

Materials:
Handout 24:2 – Focus on Music

Instructions:
In class, your instructor will play portions of slower movements of the classical composers and the Instrumental/New Age music. You will follow along using Handout 24:2 – Focus on Music.

Handout 24:2 - Focus on Music

Throughout our discussion today, either with your eyes open or closed, listen to each of the pieces of music. Describe the images that come to mind, the feelings that you have, and the mood in which you sense yourself as you listen to each song.

	Author	Title	Feelings, sensations, images, moods and thoughts evoked by song
1			
2			
3			
4			
5			
6			
7			
8			
9			
10			
11			
12			
13			
14			
15			

RELATED WEBSITES

Music Therapy Makes a Difference
Thorough overview of music therapy as it has been used to treat a variety of conditions.
http://www.musictherapy.org/

Humor: An Antidote for Stress
Excellent overview of humor as a way of managing stress.
http://www.jesthealth.com/artantistress.html

Top 5 Stress Management Mistakes
Consider these as ineffective (but commonly used) ways to deal with stressful situations.
http://stress.about.com/cs/copingskills/a/mistakes.htm

ADDITIONAL ACTIVITY - STRESS MANAGEMENT FOR LIFE CONTRACT

Objectives: The purpose of this activity is to provide you with an opportunity to develop a plan for incorporating stress prevention and stress management techniques into your daily life.

Materials needed: Handout - Stress Management for Life Contract

Description of Activity: The true value of a stress management course comes not just in learning the content, but in applying the content for improved quality of life through stress management and prevention. The focus of your book is on stress management for life (not just for the semester).

Complete the Stress Management for Life Contract and bring it to the next class. Start by setting goals for the next 8 weeks. At that time you can reassess your goals. Think about how you can develop a plan to incorporate stress management and prevention techniques into your daily routine for a lifetime of better health.

STRESS MANAGEMENT FOR LIFE CONTRACT

I, _____, agree to practice the following stress management strategies with the understanding that I will enhance my health and quality of life. I commit myself to the following goals for the next _____ weeks. This agreement with myself will be in effect from _____ to _____. At that time I will reassess my goals.

The two specific stress management goals I have set for myself are (write your goals in the SMART format; Specific, Measurable, Action-oriented, Realistic, and Time-based):

Goal #1_____

_____

_____

Goal #2_____

_____

_____

I realize I may sabotage my plans by:_____

_____

_____

So, I will avoid this by:_____

_____

_____

Family members and friends who will assist me in reaching my goals are:_____

_____

The payoffs I will realize by fulfilling my goals are:_____

_____

_____

My reward for keeping this contract will be:_____

_____

Signed: _____   Date:_____

Witness: _____